The Future of Healthcare for Seniors

George O. Obikoya

Table of Content

Executive Summary

Healthcare systems worldwide are under financial strain. With health spending increasing and in some instances with no corresponding improvement in healthcare delivery, the pressure is on from the public for health systems not only to justify their enormous expenditures, but also to curtail them. Yet, the public is becoming an increasingly suave healthcare consumer, demanding accessibility to qualitative healthcare at affordable costs. However, the expectation of qualitative health service delivery under budgetary constraints might prove too daunting for many if not all health systems, and could pose a significant challenge to their survivability, let alone, profitability, in the long term. The current financial burden on health services might even worsen with time for a variety of reasons, in developed countries, for example, because of the projected increase in the number of seniors with increasing longevity and their population aging. With seniors, the most intensive users of health services and with many of them, having one or more chronic illnesses, that this increase in their population could further swell health spending, and significantly too, is hardly disputable. What remains contentious is what we could do to prevent the possible collapse of health systems, were something not done to curtail soaring healthcare costs. This e-book is an attempt to address this issue from a healthcare information and communications technologies perspective. It advances the position that healthcare delivery is a conglomeration of processes linking interrelated systems, working individually, and in tandem to produce the outcome, namely, healthcare delivery, incurring transaction costs along the way, the quality of this outcome dependent on the efficiency and effectiveness of the processes.

The e-book highlights the need for health systems to appreciate the underlying

process flaws that invariably manifest in the problems that threaten their abilities to achieve the dual objectives of qualitative yet affordable healthcare delivery. It exemplifies the need to decompose these processes in order to determine the flaws and to rectify them, and argues for the widespread implementation and utilization of healthcare ICT as the most efficient and cost-effective means for so doing. There is increasing research evidence of the benefits that these technologies offer in improving the quality of healthcare delivery and reducing its costs. By analyzing such evidence in-depth, and relating these analyses to developments in health systems in different parts of the world, the e-book also attempts to underscore the universality of process interplay in healthcare delivery and by extension, that of the key role that health information and communications technologies could play in correcting anomalous processes, hence improving outcome quality. It also emphasizes the importance of process decomposition as an engine for the exposition that could result in further decomposition, revealing new and possibly cryptic processes whose improvement would further improve process and outcome quality, sine qua non for the necessary continuous quality improvement contingent upon the changes that our inherently dynamic health systems engender.

There could be no gainsaying the value of healthcare ICT to the future of health

services provision to not only our seniors but also the entire citizenry. Now is when we should call on one another to initiate new and step-up current efforts to promote the pervasive deployment of the technologies that could ensure that our health systems not only continue to provide the services our peoples expect them to, and even better, but also prepare adequately to meet the challenges of the future. This e-book hopes to add a voice to this call.

Introduction

Healthcare provision for seniors is could easily become the albatross of health

service systems in the developed countries in the next five years when the first set of baby-boomers become seniors. With the population in these countries aging as life expectancy increases, the number of seniors is going to increase steadily and coupled with low-birth rates could mean that these countries would have a preponderance of the elderly. This in itself is not necessarily a bad thing, witness the many that now delay retirement, or return to work after retirement, full time or part time. In fact, barring the operations of another subtle but significant factor in the labor market, ageism, increasingly many more seniors would be re-joining the labor force in the years ahead, many highly skilled, and in particular with the expertise and knowledge that these countries increasingly service-based economies need, and of which in the main increasingly lack enough. In fact, some of this expertise is in healthcare fields. Even now, with healthcare systems in many countries guzzling significant portions of their gross Domestic Products (GDP,) concerns are already fever pitched, and understandably. In many of these countries, not only are healthcare expenditures skyrocketing, some do not think that the health system is delivery the qualitative healthcare to justify such expenses. At the end of the day, the taxpayer is short-changed, and compromised, as far as health goes. What's more, the unhealthier the peoples are, the costlier it is to run the health system. Thus, the health system winds up in a vicious circle whose result would unlikely favor anyone and, probably spell disaster for the country. It is not difficult to see for example how the country's productivity, sports, businesses, roads, education, security systems, and indeed, its entire economy could collapse with its population unhealthy, the ravaged economies that the HIV/AIDS "pandemic" left in its wake in particular in sub-Saharan Africa are obvious examples of the importance of a healthy populace. This virus, incidentally is still waxing strong across the globe, as is another, the 5HN1, reportedly showing signs lately of probably being able to hop from person to person, which if so, could signal the start of the much-dreaded avian flu pandemic. With jets able to shuttle five hundred passengers across the globe at once now in airline fleets, the interrelatedness of health systems worldwide, and the need for collaboration to stop the intercontinental spread of these and other microbes could hardly be in question. In other words, healthcare provision is not just a local enterprise it is one that increasingly requires the concerted efforts of nations working together for the betterment of humankind. Besides travel, the mobility of labor makes the intermingling of peoples from different parts of the world even more certain, as it does the chances of a variety of health problems, even if not microbes, also traveling around. This would likely put a lot of pressure of the health services of host countries particularly if such migrant laborers did not pay taxes yet utilize the host countries' health services and in fact other social services. This would further compromise health systems that are already under heavy strain, and their abilities to provide needed healthcare for seniors in particular, who are the heaviest users of these services and would likely even use them more in the years ahead. There are therefore, compelling reasons why we need to take the issues concerning the future of healthcare delivery to seniors seriously, as they essentially pertain to those critical to these health systems surviving at all as we know them today. Indeed, the earlier we start to examine ways by which we could achieve the dual objectives of qualitative healthcare delivery while simultaneously reducing healthcare costs the likelier we would be able to avert the possible collapse of our health systems under the projected increasing burden of use by an increasing number of seniors in the years ahead. There is of course no one way to solving the health problems of one country let alone for all the countries of the world. These different countries have different health issues, although there are some that are common to all. Significantly, though, the common problems, if adequately addressed seem likely to create the enabling environment to resolve the other less generic problems. These common problems pertain to the processes, and there are literally thousands of them, involved with every stage of healthcare delivery. In other words, by improving these processes, or those that need fixing, which would differ in individual countries, we could be creating the milieu for us to achieve the dual healthcare delivery objectives mentioned earlier. This book explores the issues involved with utilizing healthcare information and communications technologies (ICT), in achieving these goals, hence in preventing the possible chaos in the health systems of many countries, particularly as the number of seniors increase in the near future.

Healthcare costs constitute the central problem in many health systems, the

increase in these costs seemingly unstoppable. Our central theme in this book is that the widespread acceptance, implementation, and utilization of healthcare ICT could stop these runaway healthcare expenditures. Further, we posit that these technologies could do so without compromising the quality of healthcare delivery, and that, contrariwise, they would in the process, improve healthcare quality. That costs would feature prominently in our discussions is understable, considering that health spending in the U.S, which has the costliest health system worldwide, was roughly 14%, the U.K's just under, 8%, and Canada's just under 10% of each country's GDP in 2001. Five years later, Canada is spending over 10% of its (GDP) on healthcare, the estimated debt of U.K's National Health Service (NHS), £750m by the end of the FY2005, despite its £76bn budget. In the U.S., experts predicted the introduction of the new Medicare drug benefit in 2006 would only have a minor effect on overall health spending, but lead to a major shift in funding from private payers and

Medicaid to Medicare. This shift could increase public funding of health care beyond 50% during the same period with likely significant budgetary implications, a bleak scenario coupled with the country's overall total health spending in 2014 projected at 18.7% of the GDP, versus 15.3% in 2003. Seniors use up most of these expenses and mostly on medications and hospitalization fees. Other cost drivers are the costs of medical technologies, and recompense for healthcare professionals. With regards prescription drugs for example, many argue that the lack of effective price controls in the U.S, unlike in Europe for example, makes prescription drugs in that country sometimes thrice more expensive than they are in other developed countries. We saw the effects of these high medication costs a few years ago with seniors crossing the border en masse to Canada from the U.S to buy their medications. Yet, experts argue that the U.S is doing everyone else a favor by pharmaceutical companies being able to reap returns on their research and development investments that result in the new drugs from which they make profits off the Americans, making it possible for patients in Europe for example, and indeed elsewhere to be able to afford them. This however, as with all the other problems that plague the U.S health system, and every health system worldwide we could decompose to process problems. Could the drug companies still not invest in medications that yield equally high social returns as the new prescription medications do, at much less expense, for example moving in tandem with the shift in medical paradigms, developing products that would still increase their bottom lines? In the same vein, could improvement in other processes that contribute on the aggregate to healthcare delivery in the country not reduce the need for the high-cost prescription medications and increase that for the new lower-cost products that drug companies would now make, and market, and which many more healthcare consumers would now buy? Would this not still make pharmaceutical products affordable to all without compromising the U.S budget? Some also argue that the drugs approval process in many countries including in the U.S is lengthy and contributes significantly to the high costs of prescription medications. Could speeding up the Foods and Drugs Administration (FDA) approval process in the U.S for example, not reduce the costs of prescriptions drugs? Because these are all issues that relate to processes, should we not be keen to invest in the healthcare ICT that could help improve these processes hence reduce transaction costs? We would explore these and other issues regarding not only the U.S health system, but also the health systems in other countries in this e-book.

There is a deceleration in private sector spending on healthcare in the U.S., private spending growth down to 7.4% in 2004, versus 8.6% in 2003, and ongoing, according to some estimates, which the Medicare drug benefit would exaggerate, growth down to 3.1% in 2006. These developments would put pressure of Medicare spending growth, estimated to accelerate 2.5% points to 8.2% in 2004, the joint state and federal Medicaid spending growth, from 7.1% in 2003 to 7.9% in 2004. Decreased health spending by the private sector in the U.S reflects increasing difficulty to cope with huge health benefits they now confront, relics of post-WWII deals between major U.S. companies for example the Detroit automakers, and workers' unions, whose faces down the road these firms seemingly did not foresee. There is also increasing health spending in public funded health systems, and paradoxically, increasing private health insurance too, as some would argue, the health system sheds some of its financial burden. The private sector in the U.K is also backing off lucrative pension schemes crucial to maintaining the well-being of retirees, hence their health status. A Detroit News report on May 31, 2006 of a survey by John Bailey & Associates indicated for example that 61% of businesses in the Detroit region are contemplating future reductions to employee health benefits. The survey was of executives from 203 firms in 3 southeastern Michigan counties, 75% of the firms with less than 100 employees, 15%, 100 to 500, and 8%, over 500. The survey showed that 27% of business executives were contemplating removing health care benefits, and 86% want ed employees to pay a larger share of health care premiums. Furthermore, 75% of executives want ed smokers to pay more for premiums, and almost as many thought that firms should reward workers with healthy lifestyles. Does this survey not support the view that the private sector is increasingly weary of rising healthcare costs? The overall picture that emerges from these different health systems is increasing public health spending, which no doubt is unsustainable. These increases could in fact worsen over the years as people live longer, with increased use of health services that could ensue, but should service utilization increase or not? We would argue in this e-book that service utilization could increase but not necessarily health spending, and in fact that the appropriate deployment of healthcare ICT could reduce some types of service utilization, for example hospitalization, and increase others, for example preventive services and overall improve the quality of healthcare delivery but not its costs. A variety of issues determine the nature and prevalence of diseases, the variety of health indicators, the effectiveness and efficiency of the auxiliary processes crucial to the delivery of health services qualitatively. These various factors, some clinical, others not, operate in an intricate medley to produce a smooth running and effectiveness health system, the very outcomes that the faulty operation of any of these processes could hamper. In other words, we argue in this e-book that we need to decompose these processes in order to appreciate fully their effectiveness and efficiency or other wise, determine their specific flaws if any, in order to be able to fix and improve them using the appropriate healthcare ICT.

Medicare Part D commenced in the U.S in 2006, providing Medicare beneficiaries

with prescription drug coverage, beneficiaries able to keep receiving employer-subsidized drug coverage, qualified for Medicare financial aid in 2006, the former as we noted earlier expected to keep increasing, the latter falling. In fact, experts projected that overall prescription drug spending will increase 11.6%, 0.5% due to Medicare Part D, an added $1.0 billion in health spending. With the variety of long-term care, seniors would expect of services, there is no doubt that the country, and indeed, all other developed countries and the developing countries with an aging population, would need to focus on critically rationalizing health spending. In fact in some countries, measures for example, mandatory long-term care insurance are already in place. As we ruminate on policy and funding strategies, and other issues pertaining to meeting the healthcare needs of our seniors in the years ahead, including assuring service quality, while curtailing costs, we argue in this e-book the need for us to appreciate the transactional nature of the underlying processes that come together as what we term healthcare delivery. We also need, as noted earlier, to decompose these transactions in the different domains, clinical and otherwise, for us to be able address the processes involved adequately. Consider the issue of healthcare ICT adoption for example, a crucial part of the process improvement efforts we need to embark upon in order to achieve our dual healthcare delivery objectives of delivering qualitative health services simultaneously reducing costs yet it comprises a series of processes in itself that we need to decompose and address. In fact, it continues to pose a major challenge to our efforts to achieve our dual goals, the reasons for the healthcare industry being slow to adopt healthcare ICT, resulting in what some experts consider as much as a decade-long lag behind other information-intensive industries such as the banking industry, multitude. They include costs, concerns about privacy and confidentiality of patient information, lost productivity, lack of standards, loss of status, problems with the doctor-patient relationship, even technophobia. Others include concerns about recouping investments, or losing it altogether as regulations or technical specifications change. Again, as we have argued thus far, these issues are also breakable into their component processes, which we could address and improve using appropriately designed healthcare ICT-backed programs, the heuristics of this approach being decomposition leading to exposition, and with further decomposition, even more exposition. With process improvement the ultimate result, which with continuous evaluation would lead to an endless process improvement dynamic, we are rest assured of the continuous achievement of our dual objectives within the evolving context of the operations of these processes. We would be undertaking a complex yet rewarding exercise understanding healthcare delivery this way and endeavoring to tackle the problems that confront it now and that would in the years ahead as the population of our senior citizens increases significantly.

ICT and the Healthcare Quality Cycle

That healthcare delivery is qualitative and accessible in most countries including

many in the developed world is to recant the obvious, to which a variety of reports, commissioned by public and private organizations and the ongoing need for health reforms in many countries, attest. However, consumer satisfaction or otherwise with the health services is perhaps the most important indicator that all is or is not well with the quality of healthcare that the populace receives. According to a July 2005 Kaiser public opinion survey in the U.S., for example,[1,2] most American adults think that nurses (84%), doctors (69%) and hospitals (64%) do a "good job" serving healthcare consumers, nursing homes (35%) rank below pharmaceutical firms (43%) and just above health insurance firms (34%), and HMOs (30%) in the quality of service provision. Most also think that nursing homes provide a safe environment for people who need them (69%), but on the affordability and quality of nursing home care, 53% agree that nursing homes provide an affordable way for people to get round-the-clock care, 39% disagree, 21%, "strongly." Forty six percent of the public agree that nursing homes provide high-quality services, 42% disagree. Indeed, the public is somewhat guarded about nursing home care, twice as many adults think nursing homes make people " worse off", 12% saying that they would choose to get care in a nursing home rather than a hospital, 39%, were they to need 24-hour healthcare. The problem that the public has with nursing homes appears not to be with their staff that 68% of those surveyed think show concern for their patients' well-being. On the other hand, the public thinks that nursing homes have inadequate staffing and defective management, and that relatives of their clients are not involved enough in their care. Seventy-four percent think that nursing homes do not have enough staff, 60%, that the staffs do not have enough training, and 58% that there is substantial waste, fraud and abuse by the managers. Now, what does this say for long-term care (LTC)? Before we examine that, 30% of those surveyed indicated that they would mostly pay for LTC by insurance if they or family members were to require nursing home care, compared to 16% and 13% that preferred personal savings, or government programs for examples, Medicare/Medicaid, respectively. However, in actuality, private insurance only pays for 8% of nursing home expenses (8%), Medicaid, the major nursing home care financing, 46%. In any case, only 21% of Americans say that they have LTC insurance, the most common reason for not having one, cost (59%), although 32% never even considered LTC insurance. Forty-eight percent concede that a federal tax-credit would encourage them to buy one, but just as many that it would not. Sixty-three percent think that government is not sufficiently involved in regulating nursing home quality, 48% that these homes do not receive enough payment by the government and other insurers. Would government regulation be counter-intuitive to free-market operations in an essentially privately funded health system such as that in the U.S, or is some form of regulation actually beneficial to the smooth operations of such health systems? Is there a need to revisit remuneration policies for LTC? These again, are pertinent questions that answered, could help not only to improve the quality of care, but its perception by the clients that the health system serves. This survey also reveals that 57% of Americans do not know where to get advice and information about nursing homes if a family member needed care in one. Is this not another example of the information asymmetry that plagues the health system in general, which with the resources that progress in information technologies continue to offer us, we should be able to redress effectively and promptly? Fifty-nine percent of the interviewees indicate that they prefer to obtain information and advice, about such information from friends and family, or their doctors, 54%, than from government websites, community service agencies, books/reports, or government programs, 27%, 25%, 25%, and 23%, respectively. Does this not suggest that these personal sources need to have the information to provide in the first place? Does this not speak to the need for targeted health information delivered direct to those that need it, analyzed and contextualized, and via the most appropriate electronic format? Should seniors, and indeed, the public at large not know for example, about a new medication that could significantly change the treatment of severe anemia, and would such information not benefit the many seniors that suffer from this condition for a variety of reasons such as defective dietary regime or illness-related poor nutrition? Indeed, many with severe anemia, for example patients with beta-thalassemia, need blood transfusions from time to time, risking hemosiderosis, or an excess of iron in the blood, side effect of such transfusions that could damage liver and the heart with potentially fatal consequences. Customarily difficult to remove, with many indeed, preferring not to do so as a result, findings from an international study on deferasirox, a new drug capable of removing excess iron from the blood less onerously will appear on May 1, 2006, in Blood, the official journal of the American Society of Hematology. Patients that need regular blood transfusions will no longer have to endure perhaps a lifetime of deferoxamine use, the current method for detoxifying the system of iron, the process, the medication given by slow subcutaneous or intravenous infusion for eight to 12 hours a night over a period of five to seven days, clearly not user-friendly. Deferasirox's once-daily oral administration, the pill dissolved in water and drank each day before breakfast, on the other hand, will no doubt be more agreeable to patients. Further, the study showed Deferasirox to be just as effective as deferoxamine in patients receiving the highest doses of the drug, and tolerated well, although 11% of study participants had side effects such as skin rash, and 15%, gastrointestinal problems, such as abdominal pain, vomiting, diarrhea, and constipation. How much could we save in human and material terms with such information as this study shows targeted at those that need regular blood transmissions, or their relatives? Could it encourage more to seek treatment, hence reduce the burden of their disease on themselves, their families, and on society? Is it not time that we started to take the issue of deploying healthcare ICT in the delivery of health services to our seniors, and indeed, to all citizens seriously? Indeed, some jurisdictions in the U.S. are already doing just that. According to the *San Francisco Chronicle*, of April 26, 2006, The San Francisco Department of Public Health has started sending safer sex advice via cell phone text messages targeted at young people who request it. The campaign will cost just $2,500 a month. San Francisco is the first U.S. city to implement such a program. The city lately recorded higher sexually transmitted infection rates among young people. For example, in 2005, the city had a 100% rise in the prevalence of gonorrhea among black teens. A similar campaign is ongoing in London, targeted at youths, aged 12 to 24 years. By sending for example the text message "sexinfo" to one of two phone numbers set up by the health department, the system will send a reply back to the inquirer asking him/her to choose one of several categories that matches the question. The language of the message is teen-friendly, and there are options for example, what the person should do if a condom broke and advice on dealing with "pressures" to have sex. The text messaging process is brief, just about a minute or two, users also given a phone number they could call for more information. According to Jacqueline McCright, community-based STD services manager at the health department, "We wanted to design a program that would reach young people with the technology they use most often," adding", Most youth get their information from their friends. ... They are winging it, trying to figure it out for themselves." Some are afraid or ashamed to ask questions on the subject of sex and related issues, and many do not visit clinics for these reasons. The text message service would likely solve these problems. The health department also launched the Web site sextextsf.org that offers more information on the program. Should many more cities and indeed, countries not implement such programs for their youths and similar targeted health programs for others such as seniors, women, and children? In Alberta province, Canada persons aged 15 to 24 years constituted 33% of all ER visits and hospitalization for self-harm in 2003/04, and approximately 24,000 young people aged 13 to 17 years visited a physician for mental health related problems during the same period. Would the province go wrong to institute preventive programs targeted at young people, for example to help them deal with potentially stressful life transitions and events? What role could healthcare ICT play in the design and delivery of such programs, and what cost-benefits might these technologies offer in the bargain, as the San Francisco example shows? Should we indeed not extrapolate this approach to tackling health problems in general, many of which the scope for preventive efforts is impressive? For example, the National Institute of Nursing Research and the National Library of Medicine of the National Institutes of Health, as well as the Rutgers Busch Biomedical Research grant are collaborating in funding a study to examine the effectiveness of computerized tailored video health promotion messages as an approach to reduce HIV risk behavior. Based on information gathered and analyzed from focus groups with women in public housing developments and other locations in Newark and Jersey City, Dr. Rachel Jones, assistant professor at Rutgers College of Nursing, has developed an urban soap opera type video vignettes for hand-held computers aimed at reducing young women's HIV sexual risk behavior. With heterosexual transmission accounting for 79% of HIV infection in women, and whereas African-American and Latina women together represent about 25% of all women in the United States, they account for 83% of AIDS diagnosis reported in 2003, and whereas HIV/AIDS and other sexually transmitted diseases not exclusive to the young, we no doubt need such targeted education efforts. Indeed, according to Dr Jones, "HIV/AIDS among women is one of the most pressing public health problems in Newark, Jersey City and the surrounding communities· ·This is a preventable disease and we want to find out if these video vignettes, with their stories and characters, will change their views or attitudes about unprotected sex." We should indeed focus more on such creative, targeted, and contextualized healthcare ICT-based, health information dissemination, if we were to enhance our chances of achieving the set health-education goals. The vignettes that Dr. Jones developed for example have stories that students and graduates of The Department of Visual and Performing Arts at Rutgers-Newark, among others perform. The HIV risk reduction message, based on the science of HIV risk and women's wisdom shared in the focus groups, communicated as each actor revisits high-risk scenes and this time acts to reduce HIV risk will most likely inspire interest in viewers imbibing the message. Part of the education process includes a post-viewing, discussion with participants, who fill out a form for their recommendations for improvements to the video vignettes this feedback producers will incorporate in future editions of the vignettes. Now, is this process not likely to make the vignettes even more contextualized, and culturally relevant, hence more acceptable to many more viewers, increasing the prospects of the message's acceptance? Dr Jones will pilot test the videos on hand-held computers with women, between 18 and 29 years old, in Newark and Jersey City in May 2006$_2$. It is clear that we have to continue to find novel ways to make health educat ion campaigns work.

There is no doubt that healthcare ICT offers us a wide range of options in achieving

this goal, and cost-effectively too. Consider also how the following developments in healthcare ICT research could affect the quality of lives of people with mobility or cognitive impairments, which many seniors even those not in nursing homes have for example. European researchers in the IST-funded ASK-IT project are developing a new software platform in association with major telecom industry players providing a holistic and integrated way to guided movement between locations. Billed for completion in December 2008, researchers are working on ASK-IT, to develop a standard ontological framework (using XML) they plan to publish on the World Wide Web (WWW) by June 2006, and to which more than 80 content providers, such as major telecom carriers, city municipalities and chambers of commerce, have already acquiesced. The ASK-IT platform has two components, the first, minute user-programmable extra software on a latest-generation mobile phone or Personal Digital Assistant (PDA). This part will have all the data and information about the individual s personal needs and preferences, for examples information about cognitive, sight, and hearing impairment and wheelchair use. The other component is a web service containing a set of data that conform to the ASK-IT universal ontology, the connotation, and associations of terms and concepts, including about local facilities and services dynamically linkable to other local information and service provider databases. ASK-IT, which enables users to read signs and find their way around in different locations with different languages, is currently undergoing databases developments in eight pilot sites in Europe, namely, Budapest in Romania, The Hague (The Netherlands), Genoa (Italy), Helsinki (Finland), Madrid (Spain), Newcastle in the UK, Nuremburg (Germany) and Thessaloniki (Greece), demonstrations billed to commence in 2007. Would this project for example not help improve the quality of life of seniors, enabling them to move more freely, even within their own countries, for example, to holiday in Quebec from Saskatoon, or even an English-speaking wheelchair-bound senior in New York to shop in parts of the city with predominantly non-English-speaking New Yorkers, and vice versa? Managed collaboratively by a motley of typically ten organizations, including private companies, to local governments, and Universities, lead partners variable with each location, does this project not demonstrate the potential of such intersectoral alliances in producing innovative healthcare ICT, and why they need encouraging? Do the variations in composition and leadership and these alliances not indicate the need for flexibility in developing business models for healthcare ICT to ensure its alignment with the peculiarities of each site including the availability of required management and technical expertise? There is no doubt about the prospects for improving the care of seniors in future with more of such valuable healthcare ICT available for their use, including in healthcare delivery, in particular with the increasing emphasis on domiciliary and ambulatory care. According to Dr Angelos Bekiaris of the Center for Research and Technology in Athens, in an IST-Results report, the project s technical manager, the ASK-IT system works in real-time, via the person s personal mobile communications device, and 'Say I m a wheelchair user traveling from home to Sweden. At home, I will plan the trip, and the system will know that I am a wheelchair user and query information about hotels with suitable access. I need to know how to reach the airport so the system provides multimodal transport information depending on my preferences. If I am traveling by bus, for example it makes recommendations based on the availability of suitable wheelchair ramps. If I am traveling by car, it will recommend parking where wheelchair access is available." He further adds, "Inside the bus it works with the bus routing system, so can tell you when to disembark for example. In the car, it will link via Bluetooth with the in-car navigation system. Once inside the airport, the system links with airport wireless networks to guide you to the departure gate. "The system uses GSM's positioning resources, and the GPS satellite system to figure someone's location, data and information it then boosts with the resources of the Russian EGNOS GPS network to offer increased location precision to within a meter. With users able to program their device to seek, book, and pay for information on added-value services online, the system is no doubt not only robust, but also versatile. It is indeed, one that experts deem only Galileo coming online in 2008 will perhaps surpass in excellence. The researchers note that these features use standard software now under development and built-in into new-generation mobile phones and PDAs, with the collaboration of such firms as Siemens (Project Coordinator), Microsoft, Alcatel, Nokia, among others. They also note the contribution to the project of an earlier one, IMAGINE-IT, specifically providing many of the modules required to secure seamless travel-mode integration, and to add the framework special user profiles support. According to Dr Angelos Bekiaris, "The result will be a user-programmable service that will be a radical improvement on what has gone before, for general users as well as those with impairments". He also notes, "The information that is available now is so generic that most people don't bother with it. But we are developing a basis for a wealth of information that will be much more useful, because the user's access device can be personalized with his or her own preferences. And it will be dynamic, if service breaks down or are unavailable, your device will be able to seek out alternatives, all in real-time." There is no doubt that this product will gain increasing use in healthcare delivery particularly to seniors and those with disabilities in the near future. Would anyone likely disagree that we should already start musing over the health of baby-boomers post 2011, just five years away? Consider the following findings from the 2003 California Health Interview Survey regarding chronic health conditions in the state. The survey, which the California Healthcare Foundation (CHCF) funded, and which offers information that counties and local health systems could use to note areas with high rates of chronic conditions, hence in program planning and resource optimization, has data and information on disease prevalence, and on other important features of healthcare services in the state such as Medi-Cal enrollment. The report also touches on health services access-indicators, and on the barriers to access to care. The report shows that in 2003, 11.5 million or 45.2% aged 18 years or above had one or more chronic health condition, and over six million adults age 18 or older (23.5 percent) had high blood pressure, almost 50% of the state's 1.7 million adults diagnosed with heart disease, 65years or older. About 40% of adults with "fair", or "poor" health saw a doctor six or more times, and of those with better health, only

14.6%, 60% of the former, low income individuals. About 1.6 million adults had diabetes, and a third of Californians (32.1%) had one or more problems accessing health services or lacking a usual source of care during the same period according to the report. Close to half, 44.7% of adults had one or more potential barriers to accessing health services for example, low income, lack of insurance, and difficulty speaking English. This report raises important questions regarding the quality of health services provision, disease prevalence rates, indicators of health and disease outcomes, and access to health services. The answers to the questions raised would no doubt help in understanding better the contributions of chronic health conditions to the burden of diseases in various domains, for example, to the individuals with these conditions, their families and to society. Chronic diseases for example cause 1.7 million deaths in the U.S. annually and contribute to about 75% of the country's annual healthcare costs4. These diseases, many of which are preventable, are also the major causes of deaths in California, as they indeed, are in many other U.S. st ates, and in most of the developed world. These diseases, even when established, are also ambulatory/domiciliary sensitive, and manageable successfully with excellent monitoring and treatment outside the hospital, which healthcare ICT appropriately deployed could help achieve much cheaper than treated in hospital settings. Understanding why for example, Los Angeles Service Planning Area (LA SPA) South, Madera County, lake/Mendocino county group, Kern County, and Colusa/Glenn county group, had the highest prevalence rates of any of these chronic conditions, namely high blood pressure, diabetes, asthma, and heart disease would yield more valuable and actionable information than the rates in themselves. So would exploring the reasons for the difficulty accessing health services by certain groups and in certain counties help in more appropriate policy formulation and service planning. Should other states in the U.S, and provinces, in Canada, and other similar jurisdictions not engage in such efforts to understand better the status of their health services in a dispassionate, matter-of-factly manner? Indeed, this is the case as the following example of Ontario, Canada shows. A recent report by the Ontario Health Quality Council (OHQC), an independent agency established as a component of the *Commitment to the Future of Medicare Act, 2004*, which received Royal Assent on June 17, 2004₁. Established on September 25, 2005, the Council's mandate is to monitor the healthcare system and report annually to Ontarians regarding accessibility to Medicare and related health resources. It also monitors population health status, and health system outcomes, all in an effort to promote quality improvement and accountability. According to the Council, its first report examines, "attributes of a high performing health system, performance indicators to measure these attributes, understanding and improving access to health care". It also examines "getting the right number and mix of people working in health care, spreading the use of proven knowledge and best practice, transforming delivery of health services, and using e-health to transform Ontario's health system". According to report released on April 26, 2006, and available at the Council's website, OHQC recognizes electronic health records (EHR) for all patients, health information management-systems, and telehealth, together known as e-health, as the key facilitators for quality improvements in the health care system. The Council considered the attributes that Ontarians expect of their health system namely: safety, effectiveness, patient-centeredness, accessibility, efficiency, equitability, and integration, also appropriate resource, and focus on population health and indicators for measuring them. According to its chair, Ray Hession, "Ontario's health system is performing well in a number of areas .But in some respects, the system needs more work". He adds, "We have found that inadequate information is limiting our ability to continuously improve quality, monitor performance and report on it'''" The chairperson also emphasized the Council s conviction that investing in e-health will do the most to improve each of the attributes of such as high-performing health system as Ontarians expect to have. According to Hession, "We concluded that the key enabler for health system improvements is e-health'''.The implementation of e-health in Ontario requires a clear plan, appropriate governance, and requisite funding." One cannot put perhaps the most important requirement for the success of any e-health program more succinctly. Consider the point the chairperson made for example, about the health system essentially lacking adequate information to assist the Council in reliably measuring the indicators of the system's performance, numerical measures of progress toward set goals, regarding the attributes of a high-performing health system that Ontarians seek. Does it not speak to the importance of healthcare ICT in other domains of health service delivery, namely in the administration, finance, and general management domains? Could healthcare ICT therefore not help address some of the administrative and management issues that the Kaiser Opinion survey raised about LTC mentioned earlier? Would the implementation of these technologies in these areas for the improvement of specific processes that would on the aggregate contribute toward the realization of measurable indicators for performance improvements in the domains relative to the attributes mentioned earlier not be more rational with proper planning? Would such planning not in fact enhance the chances of these technologies being more efficient and cost-effective, and indeed, yield returns on investments (ROI)? Does the fact that these technologies by improving the quality of the processes required to actualize goals in these non-clinical domains create the enabling milieu for clinical process improvement, for example buoying supply chain processes thus ensuring continuous availability of required medical equipments and supplies, not speak to their being indeed crucial to the success of contemporary health systems? True to its vision of being "a trusted, independent voice dedicated to improving the health and healthcare of all Ontarians", the Council also highlighted the deficiencies in the province's health system. With regard safety for example, while the Council found evidence for a progressive lessening of the number of patients that break bones while in an acute care hospital, or develop skin ulcers, while in a chronic care hospital, it recommends a zero tolerance for preventable adverse events. The Council noted that a cross-Canada study suggests there were likely about 32,000 preventable adverse events in Ontario's Hospitals in 2004, and regretted its inability to count these events accurately because of the lack of health information systems to track them accurately in the province. As the Council rightly noted, "This makes it difficult to determine how to reduce or eliminate adverse events." The Council also noted that Ontario's Patient Safety Task Force is to report in the spring of 2006 with possibilities for continuing improvements in care and safety that the Council could monitor in future, and hoped that with improvement in patient safety measurement would be fewer medication errors and other injurious events.

The Council's observations on safety suggest the need for further efforts at integrating the various adverse events reporting agencies currently operating in the country. There is no doubt about the potential wealth of data and information regarding various aspects of adverse events reporting that these agencies have in their databases, including regarding Ontario. Health Canada is the federal regulatory authority for the safety, efficacy, and quality of therapeutic products used in Canada pursuant to the *Food and Drugs Act (F&DA.)* Indeed, as was the case involving imported human cells, tissues and organs (CTO), with the ban on tissues from CryoLife, Inc., pursuant to a major safety problem reported to the U.S. Food and Drug Administration (USFDA), the country's health authorities take safety issues seriously. Indeed, the Krever Inquiry report of 1997 and the Performance Review of Canadian Blood Services of 2002 both resolved that voluntary compliance should not be an option in regulatory frameworks because it provides inadequate oversight and that a federal regulatory framework was required. Specific safety standards, compliance monitoring and enforcement activities, and adverse event reporting are all essential activities for ensuring the safety of health products. For example, the Canadian Standards Association (CSA) published the national Safety Standards for CTO in 2004, standards, including adverse events reporting, that are measurable, hence could reveal valuable information on compliance with safety levels. Canada not only has regulations for adverse event monitoring for the purpose of regulation under the *Food and Drug Regulations,* but also regarding epidemiological comprehensive surveillance by the Public Health Agency of Canada (PHAC) for tracking, monitoring, and evaluating the outbreak of infectious diseases and adverse outcomes. It is important for the country to continue to gather, collate, store, analyze and interpret reported data on adverse events in order to enhance its surveillance system's capability regarding risk detection, and the provision of apposite data for risk management decision making. Provincial/territorial laws mandate the reporting of infectious diseases for example, with variations in the lists across jurisdictions. However, in most cases, the doctor that made the diagnosis of an infectious disease must submit a report under these laws in a timely manner, even if of suspected cases rather than waiting to confirm the diagnosis, to local health authorities. The health authorities pass the reports on to the appropriate provincial/territorial authority if the case was reportable case based on stipulated criteria, with cross-province information sharing possible per agreements among these provinces/territories. These processes clearly highlight the presence of veritable databases in these jurisdictions, and underscore the need for the implementation of the appropriate, and interoperable healthcare ICT for the seamless communication and sharing of this information, for example not just between provinces, but within provinces and between provincial and federal agencies. Canadian Adverse Drug Reaction Information System (CADRIS) for example monitors adverse drug reactions in drugs approved for the Canadian market. Provincial/territorial health authorities should not only be able to access these data but should also have seamless electronic connection with them to facilitate data and information sharing, and database update with new data and information from the field. In fact, the Canadian Broadcasting Corporation (CBC) acquired Canada's Adverse Drug Reaction Database, which it published online, from Health Canada. This database, which uses data collected from 1965 to Sept. 30, 2003, has information from all adverse drug reaction (ADR) reports currently held in Health Canada's CADRIS database, although not all data and information contained in CADRIS, Health Canada, for example, withholding certain information in compliance with the country's privacy laws6. The Council also addressed the other attributes that Ontarians wish for their health system namely, that it should be effective, accessible, efficient, equitable, integrated, appropriately resourced, and focused on population health, including required measures for improving on the status quo, and indeed, recommendations for future goals. For examples, the Council mentioned that according to the Canadian Community Health Survey, close to 1 million Ontarians do not have access to a regular family doctor, which would likely keep them from receiving preventive care, for example screening and immunizations, and make it harder to see specialists. The Council also noted the disparity in access to care based on income levels, among others, for examples the poor, immigrants, aboriginals, and rural residents having more difficulties accessing care. According to the report, Ontarians with higher incomes that have chest pain receive quicker hospital treatment than their less financially endowed counterparts, which latter in fact tend to be more ill, that women are twice as likely to receive a prescription for a tranquilizer as men are. The report indicated that just 4% of Ontario hospitals have stroke units, proven to decrease death rates and pricey hospitalizations. The report also observed that women that suffer from heart disease are less likely to receive diagnostic tests and surgery, and that just 50% persons newly diagnosed with diabetes mellitus receive an eye test within one year to prevent what may result in blindness, an examination preferably done when diagnosed. Another pertinent observation in the report was that individuals that live in the north of the province access heart procedures, hip and knee replacements and cataract and cancer surgeries easier than those in the south do, although the latter are, on the average healthier, and live longer. There is no doubt about the important role that healthcare ICT could play in resolving many of these issues, which makes the Council s assertion of the need for e-Health expected. However, there is likely none also that reports by organizations such as Ontario Health Quality Council give us an indication of the state and quality of healthcare delivery, but they also point in the direction we should focus regarding improving the quality of health services delivery. The questions brought up earlier, regarding access to care, and the importance of geographical, demographic, and other issues in determining diseases prevalence, and of the indicators of health and disease outcomes apply to these findings from Ontario too. In other words, we also need to interpret the findings of such reports appropriately for us to apply them effectively in tackling the healthcare delivery issues that they raise. Indeed, this would facilitate the determination of needs areas for healthcare ICT implementation, the specific technologies most appropriate to solving the identified problems cost-effectively, hence a more rational healthcare ICT deployment, and ultimately, better chances of realizing ample returns on the investments in these technologies. As mentioned in our discussion on the Kaiser Opinion survey earlier, the remuneration of healthcare professionals has close ties with quality improvement efforts regarding health services delivery. Yet, these are thorny issues whose resolution continues to be elusive even as debates on the best approaches to resolving the issues continue unabated. Consider the concept of pay-for-performance, for example, in which an increasing number of physicians in the U.S now take part, receiving inducement bonus payments for accomplishing healthcare-delivery quality targets. The question remains though whether this model would help us achieve our dual objectives of improving healthcare delivery while simultaneously reducing healthcare costs, considering the clearly-unsustainable, ever-increasing healthcare costs that many countries including in the developed world seem determined, and understandably so, to curtail. The connection between promoting qualitative healthcare delivery and remuneration transcends costs issues though. The U.S. Institute of Medicine (IOM) of the National Academies released a report in 1999 titled To Err is Human: Building a Safer Health System7, which showed strikingly high rates of medical errors resulting in avoidable agony, disability, and death. Besides the value proposition by the medical profession to its clients to do no harm, which puts the onus on its members to ensure that they deliver on their promise, how could anyone not shudder at the thought of medical errors killing some 44,000 people in U.S. hospitals annually according to one study, and by another's estimates, 98,000. As the report noted, even just on account of the findings of the former study, more people died from medical mistakes annually than from highway accidents, breast cancer, or AIDS. The report, which noted that medical errors occurred in not only hospitals but in other healthcare settings, for examples, day-surgery and outpatient clinics, retail pharmacies, nursing homes, and home care, emphasized that the need to reduce medical errors will necessitate significant changes in the health system including mandatory reporting requirements. Other notable comments by the Committee that wrote the report included that expertise existed to prevent errors, and it recommended a minimum goal of 50% reduction in error rates in five years. The report noted that most medical errors were not due to individual recklessness, but from basic flaws in the organization of the health system, and the committee recommended a four-part plan aimed at creating both financial and regulatory incentives that will promote safer healthcare delivery. It also emphasized evaluating the recommendations after five years to assess progress in improving safety of the health system. The IOM released another report in 2001 titled, Crossing the Quality Chasm: A New Health System for the 21st Century8, prepared by the committee on the Quality of Health Care in America. The report called for urgent action to redesign the U.S health system in order to effect the fundamental changes necessary to close the quality gap. As with the health the approach of the OHQC discussed earlier, although the latter, based on what Ontarians stipulated that they wanted their health system to be, the IOM report offered a set of performance expectations for the C21st health care system. It also recommended a set of 10 new rules to guide patient-clinician relationships, major steps to promote evidence-based practice and reinforce healthcare ICT, as did the 1999 report, the need for an organizing framework to better align incentives inherent in payment and accountability with quality improvement.

Six years after the release of the first IOM, a study appeared in the December 04, 2005 edition of the Journal of the American Medical Association that indicated that there was some improvement in hospital safety systems in the U.S. but that the improvements fell short of the IOM recommendations[9]. The researchers constructed seven variables to evaluate patient safety in the hospitals they studied. The variables included physician order entry (CPOE) systems; computerized test results and appraisal of adverse effects; specific patient safety policies; data use in patient safety programs; drug storage, administration, and safety procedures followed; mode of handling adverse event/error reporting; prevention policies and root cause analysis, their results: modest improvement. Thus, 74% of hospitals had a written safety plan, almost 9%, none. Most hospitals had medication safety systems, only 3% had fully implemented CPOE. According to Dr. Longo, one of the researchers, "We were very surprised; we expected to see more dramatic changes" "These results should act as a reminder to the hospital community and the public at large that the IOM report results have not been fully implemented". Dr. Longo adds, "Hospitals will be able to see where they need to make improvements because we have comprehensively listed all the safety systems that a hospital must have". This report calls attention to the fact that there are systematic problems. We are not talking about bad apples." Indeed, these words echoed those of the Committee that wrote the 2001 IOM report, the problems of the U.S. health system, essentially systematic, rather than individual-based, perhaps one dare adds, in the main. In other words, there is no doubt about the multifactorial roots of the problems confronting the U.S. health system, even if most were inherent in the system. Before we proceed with our discussion on improving t he quality of health systems, in the U.S., and elsewhere, it might be apt to recap the basic objectives of such quality improvement endeavors. Primarily, improving the quality of healthcare delivery will improve the health overall, of any country's peoples. This would improve the country's productivity and by extension, prosperity. Indeed, such prosperity will likely be sustainable, particularly if we paid attention to the characteristics of the health system that meet the requirements of the peoples. We must also, however, pay attention to the health needs of the peoples as scientifically determined, the resources available for health spending, and a variety of other factors contextual to the country, and in keeping with its quest for good relations with it s neighbors, and the comity of nations. In addition, a healthy nation will not keep spending disproportionate ratios of its resources on health, limiting resources to cater for other important tasks such as maintaining law and order, education, and social services, perhaps even ending up increasing taxes in order to meet these obligations. Companies will no longer be reeling under the burden of health benefits, some increasingly uncompetitive hence losing market share precipitously, forcing them to lay-off thousands of their employees. A qualitative health system will likely reduce the chances of individuals' illnesses lingering on due to substandard healthcare, further increasing the burden of diseases in a variety of ways. Such a system if in place would reduce the growing concerns over the future of healthcare for our seniors and for baby-boomers who will turn seniors in just five years.

How crucial is the issue of remuneration in regard quality improvement in

healthcare delivery? Will pay-for-performance, a.k.a (P4P), or pay-for-quality, or pay-for-reporting, which assumes that doctors will provide better care if we offered them financial incentives for example help improve quality? Many believe it would but not all. Some in the latter category for example worry that the incentive might be going into the wrong hands, considering the complexities of patient care. In other words, pay-for-performance has to be able to determine whom among the various doctors and specialists responsible for achieving expected results/outcomes, which by the way, we ought to know in advance, for a specific health problem. They contend that it is not difficult to see for example, the difficulty in doing that where a number of doctors, for the GP, the general surgeon, the urologic surgeon, the ophthalmologist, and the orthopedic surgeon, all of who may the care of patient X with say diabetes may involve. Such appraisal of who to pay for what performance would clearly even be more problematic in the case of say a senior with a multiplicity of health problems, with the possibility of the correctness or lack thereof of the diagnoses, crucial to offering the appropriate treatments, both in the short and long-terms. Proponents however, argue that we could use algorithms for both diagnosis and treatment based on evidence, whose generalized use healthcare ICT could enable and facilitate. Thus, they contend that what we need to do is to encourage doctors to implement these technologies, and promote healthcare ICT diffusion in a concerted effort toward an e-Health milieu, in as broad a sense of the term, as practicable. It is not enough for example, for a doctor in an ER in a remote hospital confronted with a patient he/she diagnosed with stroke to know that he/she needs to give the patient tissue plasminogen activator (t-PA). The doctor also ought to be able to seek and obtain expert opinion via say telehealth, if lacking the experience in the use of this and other medications or medical procedures, help that could save the lives of many of his/patients. How could the ER doctor obtain such help without such technologies in place? Indeed, such technologies could enable the ER learn other skills from experts that his/her particular hospital lack, or doctors in general to acquire new knowledge and skills. Consider for example the results of a new study published in the May 02, 2006 edition of the Journal of the American College of Cardiology that Cardiology residents could learn to perform precarious catheterizations such as carotid angiography on a virtual patient simulator, rather than on real patients. Twenty interventional cardiologists participating in the Emory NeuroAnatomy Carotid Training program had an instructional course on carotid angiography after which they performed five serial simulated carotid angiograms on the Vascular Interventional System Training (VIST) VR simulator[10]. They made fewer mistakes, performed the virtual procedure in less time, and subjected their virtual patient to less X-ray imaging and smaller doses of parenteral contrast agent during the last versus the first run. The researchers cautioned that, their findings pertained to just a specific model of simulator, the Procedicus Vascular Interventional System Trainer (VIST) that Mentice AB in Gothenburg, Sweden developed, and that studying others would be necessary to individually before use to measure trainee doctors performance. Nonetheless, there is no doubt about the potential benefits of these and other technologies in training healthcare professionals even off educational campuses, hence helping to alleviate the problems of shortage of personnel in various professional cadres, an important hindrance to accessibility to care, for example, and in general in achieving our goals of qualitative healthcare services for all. In this study, trainees using the simulator utilize catheter controls similar to those used in actual procedures on one end, the other end of the catheters hooked to sensors that feed movement data into a computer, enabling the trainee to "feel" realistically, a sensation of movement of the "catheter". He/she is also able to view the "tips" progress on a monitor image akin to the fluoroscope X-ray image they would view in an actual procedure. Carotid angiography, and the related procedure of carotid stenting, is a technically difficult, as anyone would imagine maneuvering a slender catheter through blood vessels into a carotid artery in the neck would be. The risks intrinsic in the procedure this necessarily place a restriction on the number of experts available to conduct this otherwise valuable procedure. According to one of the researchers, Dr Cates, "In carotid angiography, where we are introducing catheters into the blood vessels that feed the brain. If a little piece of material breaks off or you do it incorrectly and knock a piece of blood clot or atherosclerotic plaque off the artery while you are putting the catheter in, it goes downstream and goes to the brain and causes a stroke. And that's a devastating event." Trainee Cardiologists no longer have to practice the procedure on animals, cadavers, or mechanical models as they previously did, followed by supervision as they performed the procedure on their first live patients. In addition to possibly improving treatment outcomes by these trainers, an obvious advantage in terms of quality evaluation, simulator training enables objective tracking of trainees' progress or learning curve, enabling the documentation of proficiency acquisition, and error rate reduction, rather than base certification on subjective instructors' appraisals. There is no gainsaying that relying on subjective evaluations could result in certifying not so proficient trainees, putting the lives of actual patients at risk, and compromising the quality of service delivery overall. According to Dr. Cates, "What we are seeing is a paradigm shift in the way we train physicians in procedural-based medicine ….where we are going to be able to measure the trainee's learning curve in a virtual environment…a "patient-safe" environment, and make sure the doctor has reached a level of competence before he then works on his first patient." There is no doubt that more studies to validate simulator training of healthcare professionals will surface or that more training centers will likely adopt the use of simulators in the years ahead as such studies confirm the validity of this training technique. Some experts note that with this study able to show that a simulator could not only help train doctors successfully, but that the progress in so doing are measurable objectively via a number of metrics such as contrast volume, fluoroscope time, procedure time, it has passed the first crucial test in the validation process. In future, such metrics might emerge able to tell experts from novices, or highlight various dimensions of the skills the trainee acquired, including aspects that need additional training. Furthermore, such objective evaluation of skills might even feature in the mainstream evaluation process, helping to rate doctors regarding the incentives that they receive in a pay-for-performance remuneration model for healthcare professionals. Opponents of an incentive program also argue that such incentives would compromise the doctor/patient relationship as the doctor preoccupied with meeting the "criteria" for receiving incentives would likely make such valuable clinical intercourse less of his/priority. Supporters would likely counter that except that the patient this time has his/her expectations of care, particularly if he/she had to pay for part or all of the care given. Indeed, many believe that patients' expectations of care are sophisticated, increasingly, which would likely continue considering the central position of the patient/client in contemporary healthcare delivery systems. It is therefore conceivable that pay-for-performance would in future incorporate patients' appraisal of the quality of healthcare that they received from their doctors, measures instituted for example to ensure that patients do not make such appraisals under duress, in or out of the doctors' practice. This again, underlines the need to promote healthcare ICT diffusion among all healthcare stakeholders, and this does not necessarily mean that every patient should have a computer, although it is desirable. On the other hand, patients could make such appraisals in answers to say three to five simple questions text-messaged to them on their cell phones, for example, by their health insurers, companies, or other payer agencies. They could also access the questionnaire on the

Internet site of these payers, in say a section of it that profiles the doctor, and has the required forms for sending feedbacks to the payers regarding the quality of the services the doctor provides. This and other measures for examples might be ways by which doctors and other healthcare professionals would find it necessary to implement basic healthcare ICT at least to enable them provide enough minimal services to keep them competitive, and in business. In other words, pay-for-performance might be one way to facilitate meeting the recommendations of bodies such as the IOM and OHQC, thereby improving the quality of healthcare delivery, including reducing medical errors and enhancing patient safety, not to mention, simultaneously reducing healthcare spending. Reimbursement for medical care remains topical, often coupled with other important healthcare delivery issues for examples, quality improvement, patient safety, consumer-driven healthcare, and healthcare costs. This persistence of the debate on payment reform regarding doctors, and indeed other healthcare professionals underlines the relevance of the subject to the two most important issues in contemporary healthcare delivery, namely, quality and costs. Put differently, resolving the reimbursement issues would help in achieving our dual objectives of providing all with qualitative healthcare without the payer plunged into a financial crisis. Interestingly, the Commonwealth Fund Medicare Chartbook demonstrates an opposite link between the cost of care and quality of care across the U. S. It showed that quality was highest in the lowest-cost regions and vice versaii. Thus, in Hawaii, a high-quality state, the yearly cost of care for a Medicare beneficiary was about $4000, and pre-Hurricane Katrina, the cost in Louisiana, the lowest-quality state, was $8000. Such variability of healthcare costs and quality across the country, among other reasons such as soaring healthcare costs, and increasing private sector healthcare premiums, prompt proponents of pay-for-performance to insist on the need for payers to demand value for money spent on health services. Indeed, many payers now use data that they have collected on doctors' performance to inform healthcare consumers and even guide them to doctors that provide high quality services at lower costs. The U.S. Congress appears to favor the similar concept of value-based purchasing, which would couple Medicare payment rates with quality and accountability, among others, a move echoed in the Physician Voluntary Reporting Program (PVRP) that the Centers for Medicare and Medicaid Services (CMS) introduced in 2005, which some say might constitute the basis for a later P4P program. These developments are going to require more intense efforts to encourage physicians to implement healthcare ICT, technologies which no doubt would enhance the quality of their services, and which they would need in order to demonstrate objectively that their practices meet the emerging requirements by payers for accountability and quality. With payers more likely to base physician remuneration on such objective and measurable quality improvement metrics, they will likely increasingly demand of physicians, clear evidence of value in the services that they provide for examples via efficiency, effectiveness, quality, and patent satisfaction metrics. Some aspects of physicians reimbursements will likely directly predicate on these measures in the near future, measures that will provide valuable and accessible, for example, via the World Wide Web, data, and information of physician practices to the healthcare consumer, making it possible for the consumer to make rational choices regarding the physicians that they patronize. There is no doubt, that these developments would require major attitudinal changes among many doctors, changes that would likely easier occur with their professional associations fully engaged in the complex negotiations that would likely characterize the change management process.

Private-payer pay-for-performance programs are springing up in large numbers in

countries such as the U.S, millions of patients already on board, by some estimates close to 50 million and consumer-driven health plans gaining currency just as swiftly. It is intuitive to suggest that physicians receive some sort of recognition at the end of the day for their efforts in meeting the quality standards that their clients demand. The ability of the health system to create the enabling environment for the healthcare consumer to make choices regarding their healthcare, and be more discernable regarding them, is indicative of the seriousness with which it considers healthcare quality issues. However, it would probably be disingenuous not consider the supply side in a free-market dynamic interplay of factors. Even in a publicly funded health system, part of the equation in the delivery of qualitative healthcare is some incentive for those that deliver the services. There is indeed, a biological basis for such an approach, such incentives serving to positively-reinforce performances that have led to the desired outcomes. The details of physician reimbursement reforms will vary however, from country to country depending on a variety of factors, including the levels of infrastructure, both administrative and technical available for actualizing the various components of the reform models proposed for each country. Nonetheless, efforts to continue to promote healthcare ICT diffusion need to continue apace. An example of such continuing efforts in this direction is the recent fulfillment of a campaign pledge by Mayor Michael R. Bloomberg and Department of Health and Mental Hygiene (DOHMH) Commissioner Thomas R. Frieden to New York City doctors. The announcement on April 30, 2006, that the City has appropriated $27 million to help provide 1,000 New York City Doctors with electronic health records (EHR) systems by 2008 no doubt, robustly fulfilled the pledge. In fact, an extra $13 million contributed by the community health centers participating in the program is matching the City's contribution. According to Mayor Bloomberg, "Having the right information at the right time in the right place is critical to making good decisions and to achieving quality results. This is especially true in health care. That is why we are investing $27 million to make sure every doctor in underserved communities can have the benefit of the most advanced electronic medical record technology available. New York City is already at the forefront of health information technology. Our Health Department has made great strides in health technology by requiring laboratories to report information electronically, using handheld computers for restaurant inspections, and monitoring 60,000 pieces of health information each day. Their leadership will help ensure prevention is key and that health priorities, such as tobacco control, HIV testing and treatment, and diabetes care are reflected in the design and implementation of these systems." Commissioner Frieden also notes, "Wider implementation of EHR technology will save lives... With literally thousands of patient care guidelines and tens of thousands of drug interactions, information technology is a necessity for patients and physicians. And EHRs have the potential to create millions of dollars in State Medicaid savings over time through improved prevention, which would reduce costly hospitalizations." These statements clearly highlight the points raised in our discussion thus far, that investing in healthcare information technologies would help achieve the dual objectives of providing qualitative healthcare to the populace, saving healthcare costs at the same time. Even if part of this investment involves encouraging healthcare professionals, who deliver these services to embrace and implement these technologies, as New York City has done, would it not have been worth it? Indeed, the city is promoting healthcare ICT diffusion across neighborhoods, including the poorest. This would make every neighborhood in the city a recipient of the immense benefits of these technologies in improving healthcare delivery, including enhanced quality, efficiency, and effectiveness of service delivery, and of patient safety, among others. EHRs for example could help reduce medical error rates, including in writing prescriptions, provide information to doctors at the point of care (POC) that could be crucial to management decisions, facilitate the development of disease prevention and health promotion programs, and in general increase access to qualitative care. Physicians will also be able to communicate patient information with one another streamlining patient care, and preventing duplication of efforts, thus saving healthcare costs. Healthcare professionals could use EHR to order medications, referrals, and lab tests, and to receive electronic information from pharmacists and laboratories, promptly. By offering a variety of opportunities for quality evaluation of the effectiveness of service provision, and enabling the collection of a variety of data and information, EHR also helps in elucidating the prevalence and patterns of emerging pubic health problems. New York is also planning to promote the widespread use of electronic prescribing (eRx), to over 2,000 providers that essentially see Medicaid patients, over the next three years. This is another important step by the city toward improving the quality of healthcare delivery, and its cost-effectiveness. This move will also help thwart fraud, and significantly reduce medication errors and adverse drug reactions. The city in fact is also committing funds, over $10 million to the purchase and implementation of an EHR system at its correctional facilities. The city wants to ensure that all its residents, including those in jails, receive, qualitative healthcare, the EHR also facilitating the coordination of the continuity of care delivery for inmates upon their release between correctional health and community clinics. These measures are no doubt commendable, and represent the sort of initiatives that we will likely continue to see in the efforts by healthcare stakeholders to promote the widespread implementation of healthcare ICT. The costs of implementing healthcare ICT no doubt deter many healthcare providers, particularly those in solo and small practices, but they also do even bigger healthcare establishments for example those in rural communities. However, we need to let the word out that healthcare ICT does not have to be pricey, and it is indeed, not always so. Furthermore, the more widespread the implementation of these technologies, just as everything else in the free market, the laws of supply and demand will kick in, and prices will fall. Healthcare providers could still improve the quality of their services utilizing some of the ubiquitous of these technologies, with minimal costs, such as the Internet, as the example of Isabel, a web-based clinical decision support system, shows. A recent study shows that Isabel prevents diagnostic errors and improves the quality of treatment decisions clinicians make. The study, published on May 01, 2006 in the open access journal BMC Medical Informatics and Decision Making shows that Isabel impelled pediatricians that used it to make a vital change to their diagnosis in 12.5% of cases, the cost to the doctor: just one-minute additional diagnostic time, and the gain: vastly improved diagnostic accuracy, even for difficult cases. The research was a collaborative effort between doctors at Great Ormond Street Hospital for Children, London, other U.K. hospitals, and Isabel Healthcare, UK. Seventy-six pediatricians, trainees, and final year medical students diagnosed 24 different simulated cases of varying diagnostic difficulty, on a trial website, the cases, based on real histories of children seen in hospitals prior to the study[12]. The researchers analyzed 751 cases diagnosed by 76 participants, study participants having listed their diagnosis before and after consulting Isabel. The researchers recorded the error rates, in particular of errors of omission, when participants failed to consider key diagnoses. Isabel consultation led to a major diagnostic change in 12.5% of all cases. Isabel reminded more than 50% of participants of at least one clinically significant diagnosis. The mean number of omissions for each participant decreased from 5.5 before consultation of Isabel, to 5.0 after, the likeliest diagnosis present in 67.5% and 74.7% of analyses, before and after consultation. Misdiagnosis causes most preventable medical errors, and represents more than 40% of medical malpractice claims. Understandably, it is also of key concern to patients, and other healthcare stakeholders. Misdiagnosis affects 1 in 5, and 1 in 6, of U.K, and U.S. adults, respectively according to recent surveys. Do Isabel and similar technologies not therefore offer remarkable and cost-effective opportunities to reduce the rates of misdiagnosis, the major first step in the entire treatment process, which if wrong, the other steps would follow similarly in a potentially lethal cascade? Would healthcare providers use of this simple, and inexpensive decision-support system (DSS), not help improve the quality of the services they deliver? Should part of our efforts to promote healthcare ICT diffusion not involve letting healthcare providers, particularly those in the smaller practices and in rural settings, and others that might be financially-challenged be aware of technologies such as Isabel that have the potential to improve the quality of their services, yet cost them little? Should there not in fact be mechanisms by which healthcare providers receive targeted information on such healthcare ICT issues as emerging and existing technologies, their benefits, and pricing? Could software vendors, or in fact some entrepreneurs not consider providing such services to healthcare professionals, and other interested healthcare stakeholders? Consider another example of how healthcare ICT use might in fact cost little, yet produce positive results. Computerized physician order entry (CPOE) generally seems out of reach of at least the smaller medical practices. Yet, research has shown that this technology could significantly reduce medical error rates. Some hospitals have invested substantially on this technology, and rightly expect dividends on their investments, which a new research conducted at the Cincinnati Children's Hospital Medical Center clearly shows is possible with just a simple change in the entry of verbal orders in the system that costs almost nothing. This is an exercise the study's findings indicate if implemented, reduces errors to nil. According to Dr. Michael Vossmeyer, pediatrician, and main author of the study, "By simply having the resident read back the order before he or she entered it into the computer, we reduced verbal order errors from 9.1 percent to zero" "Although this was a small study, these results are very encouraging". At this hospital, doctors conduct ward rounds inside the patient's room to foster a more family-centered encounter, with orders entered into the computer system right away, which senior doctors dictate for a resident to enter into the system. The study involved 70 such orders taken consecutively by teams on rounds, and examined for errors after the rounds, with just 9.1% error rate found, most in dosages that would not have affected safety, although they involved the intern writing down the wrong drug in two cases. The researchers also established a process of order read back involving the resident reading back the order entered prior to leaving the patient's room, to be sure it is accurate, which the senior doctor in turn additionally verifies. After starting this process, which took just a few seconds more to the visit to a patient's room, thus did not constitute a bottleneck to process flow, the researchers looked at 75 orders for errors, and found none. The researchers plan to conduct follow-up studies to determine if the findings were replicable, and the process, reliable. There is no doubt that for such a simple process to reduce medical error rates so significantly is remarkable, and that it clearly has the potential to save many lives, and increase the quality of service delivery. Efforts must no doubt continue to promote healthcare ICT diffusion, as part of the overall efforts to improve the quality of healthcare delivery. Further, and as our discussion so far indicates, the increasing sophistication of patient expectation of health service delivery, which along with a variety of other factors enable us to fashion acceptable standards of care and devise the metrics to measure them formally, create a both an ethical, and in some cases, a rational-business imperative for doctors to embrace quality. The result: a progressive and voluntary if not even expedient shift toward performance improvement, for which implementing healthcare ICT, which again, as our discussion so far shows, could help achieve, would be the next logical step. However, that these technologies could involve substantial capital outlay in some cases underscores the need for whatever we could do to encourage their adoption and implementation by healthcare providers. There is no doubt that the immense benefits derivable from improvements in the quality of healthcare delivery would permeate all domains of the health services, clinical, administrative, finance, and so on, particularly, and as previously mentioned, healthcare ICT are not necessarily restricted to clinical process improvement. With regard to the health of our seniors however, and in anticipation of the requirements on the health system of that of the baby-boomers in just five years time, our discussion on the need for improving the quality of our health services takes a new and more profound dimension. There is no doubt that there are now and would still be ample room for preventive health services regarding seniors' health and that of the baby-boomers when they become seniors. However, the fact is that we should expect to be involved with secondary and tertiary than with primary prevention in this population. In other words, much of the healthcare that our present-day seniors need, and those that baby-boomers would, when they become seniors would involve the prompt diagnosis and treatment of diseases, and the institution of measures to prevent, delay, or attenuate their long-term sequelae. The question then is where we would be providing them with these services. Treatment settings would of course vary depending on the disease in question, but there are reasons to believe that in the main, they should be in domiciliary and ambulatory settings. For one, there are quality of life (QOL) issues that we need to consider. Most persons would prefer to receive treatment in the comfort of their homes, amongst their loved ones. There is a certain psychological assurance of safety under those circumstances, and in particular with the elderly, one of perhaps expiring peacefully in their sleep, or surrounded by their family members, among others. Then there are cost issues, which would concern seniors even more, especially if they had to pay part or all their medical expenses out of pocket. Hospitalizations costs are also significant cost drivers with regard government health spending and those of other payers. Furthermore, many of the medical conditions that seniors have are chronic illnesses amenable to ambulatory and domiciliary care, made even more so, and indeed, more cost-effectively, particularly with the deployment of the appropriate healthcare ICT in the delivery of these services. Yet, it is important for the healthcare providers involved in the domiciliary/ambulatory services to have these technologies in order to use them, and as we have seen earlier, these are the very healthcare providers that often lack the financial resources, hence the will or interest in implementing these technologies. In other words, we need to intensify our efforts to encourage healthcare providers in small practices, solo practitioners, health centers in rural settings, and remote areas, and so on, to adopt, and implement healthcare ICT as part of our efforts at looking ahead to how best to meet the health services needs of our present-day and future seniors.

Promoting healthcare ICT diffusion in general is only one aspect of what we need to

do, however. There is no doubt that this would on the aggregate enhance the quality of health service provision, but would it if the technologies were themselves defective, or of poor quality? Part of our quality assurance efforts therefore should involve ensuring that the technologies we plan to use in delivering healthcare must necessarily be of high quality. This underscores why developments such as the following are positive, particularly in the context of the future of healthcare delivery to our seniors. President Bush called in April 2004 for widespread utilization of health information technology (HIT), and for electronic health records (EHRs) to be in use for most Americans by 2014. Pursuant to this call, the Office of the National Coordinator for Health Information Technology (ONCHIT) identified the private sector certification of healthcare ICT products as a major step toward the achievement of this goal. This culminated in the establishment of the Certification Commission for Healthcare Information Technology (CCHIT), launched collaboratively by the American Health Information Management Association (AHIMA), the Healthcare Information and Management Systems Society (HIMSS) and The National Alliance for Health Information Technology (Alliance) in July 2004, as a voluntary, private-sector organization to certify these products. CCHIT has been working on certification criteria and an inspection process for these technologies in three domains, namely, ambulatory EHRs, inpatient EHRs, and the networks via which they interoperate, for which it received a three contract from the Health and Human Services (HHS) in September 2005. It has completed work in the first area, the certification of EHR products for physician offices, commercial certification launched on May 3, 2006. With its final criteria for testing and certifying ambulatory EHRs out, ambulatory EHR-vendors are now free to apply for certification of their products from May 3-12, 2006, the certification fee, $28,000, will cover application, tests and a first-year certification maintenance fees, and a panel of jurors, including a practicing doctor and an IT security expert will participate in the testing. Upon passing the tests, products will receive a sticker stating the year and type of product certified, with those that failed offered a chance for retesting and appeal, announcement of the first certified healthcare ICT products billed for July 2006. The certification process even includes a 30-day public comment period and pilot tests of the system, testament to the fairness of the entire process, and its recognition of the significance of healthcare consumers, and the need to involve them in matters pertaining to the quality of healthcare delivery, and indeed all of its aspects. That there are 264 functional criteria for ambulatory EHRs, 245 of which are fully validated attests to the rigor that the certification process entails. CCHIT also aims to assist physicians in their choices of EHRs vis-à-vis the veracity of the claims of product excellence that marketing efforts invariably are all about. CCHIT will also in time, commence certification of EHRs for hospitals and other inpatient environments, and then those of the infrastructure and network components required for inter-provider data exchange. With such certification efforts proceeding unfettered, we would be ensuring that our efforts at healthcare ICT do likewise. More doctors would purchase and implement healthcare ICT that they know has the seal of approval of such credible organizations as the CCHIT, rest assured that they are buying high-quality and dependable technologies that would likely yield returns on their investments. It would be much easier to convince them to invest on these technologies, which they also know would be interoperable with those of their colleagues, and others in the healthcare-delivery value chain, with the increasing adoption by all of the technologies that have the seal of approval of the CCHIT and similar organizations in other countries. There are of course several dimensions of quality besides assuring that of the technologies we use in delivering healthcare. In fact, part of why certification is important is because it is a critical aspect of standardization, which latter is itself crucial for interoperability, which is one of the most important technical requirements for information communication and sharing. Healthcare providers could use just the health information stored in their computer systems for the management of their patients but no doubt need additional data and information, for examples lab results, to manage their patients in most instances. They would have to communicate with other members of the health team such as in the labs, the pharmacy, and in the X-Ray departments to obtain this information, something they could do much more efficiently electronically rather than by fax, or snail mail. In many cases, also, more than one physician would be involved in patient management and there would be the need for information communication and sharing among these healthcare providers, again better conducted electronically. These scenarios clearly illustrate the importance of ensuring that the technologies each of these different services and healthcare professionals use are able to integrate and communicate seamlessly. One way to ensure such interoperability is to have standards with which these technologies comply, hence the importance of certification. Making sure that the technologies whose diffusion we promote are of high quality and interoperable is going to be an ongoing process as new technologies emerge from time to time. Each country therefore needs to have the relevant agencies either in the public or private sectors or indeed and ideally in both that oversee these certification and standardization efforts. These aspects of quality assurance could actually turn out to be the most crucial in our efforts not just promote the widespread use of healthcare ICT, but also, to ensure that these technologies serve the intended dual purposes of enabling us to deliver qualitative health services to all and to curtail the ever-increasing healthcare costs many countries currently confront. These issues are going to be very important in the near future with regard to healthcare delivery to our seniors, particularly in a couple of years when present-day baby-boomers, characteristically already suave in their tastes, including for healthcare, turn 65. To underscore these points, President Bush, in a speech he gave to the American Hospital Association (AHA) on May 01, 2006, called on Congress to act to curtail increasing health costs. The President also called on hospitals to make price data for medical procedures available to the public to drive down health care costs. According to President Bush, "If we want to be the leader of the world, we must do something about'" rising health care costs. He added, "And my administration is determined to do something about it   We're asking doctors and

hospitals and other providers to post their walk-in prices to all customers"'Every hospital represented here should take action to make information on prices and quality available to all your patients. If everyone here cooperates''':., we can increase transparency without the need for legislation from the United States Congress." The President noted that Medicare would start posting price data on the Internet with effect from June 1, 2006. Healthcare ICT would help these hospitals post their pricing data for public consumption more efficiently and cost-effectively, for example via the World Wide Web, where they could actually update the prices, annotate them, and reach a wider audience rather sending the information to their clients via snail mail. However, these technologies could also make their services more cost-effective, hence their pricing more competitive. Furthermore, they could be the vehicle for distinctive value propositions that could give them a competitive edge. These issues may sound mundane but considering the direction healthcare delivery is likely heading, particularly with regard the care of our seniors and of baby-boomers when they become seniors, they are going to command the attention of hospital management boards increasingly in the near future. In a health system such as in the U.S., hospitals are going to have to justify their very existence as they face stark options, including downsizing and even closures, due to a combination of mounting debts and the redundancy of their services, as alternative, tailored, and more cost-effective ambulatory/domiciliary services emerge. Incidentally, healthcare providers that hitherto worked in these hospitals would likely be involved in these novel health services tailored to specific age groups, diseases, even gender or personal interests such as healthcare services devoted to preventing and treating diseases peculiar to pet owners, or the zoonoses. Zoonotic diseases are diseases transmissible from animals such as Lyme disease, salmonella, toxoplasmosis, rabies, and bovine spongiform encephalopathy (BSE), a.k.a. "mad cow disease". There are already healthcare providers in the U.S., Canada, the U.K., and many other developed countries that offer such specialized preventive and curative health services, and their numbers are increasing. These developments place the onus on the providers of such services, many of whom would likely be by business enterprises with health services orientation run just as its owners would the other businesses they have that may be in the energy, financial, or a non-health-related sector. Here again, we see the need to anticipate these possible developments and establish the means by which to assure the various dimensions of quality, technical, clinical, and managerial that would be necessary if we were to achieve the dual healthcare delivery goals mentioned earlier. As the President noted in his speech to the AHA mentioned earlier, price information from hospitals, along with greater use of health savings accounts, for example would mobilize market forces to lower healthcare costs. Not only will Americans that lack coverage be able to afford and have one, they will be more quality-focused in making their choices of healthcare providers, which would, in tandem with the operations of market forces, essentially mandate healthcare providers to embrace and implement the necessary quality measures to secure their competitiveness, albeit their very survival. This would likely involve implementing the necessary healthcare ICT to improve their workflow processes, and make their services more effective and efficient. As noted earlier in our discussion, the prevailing degree of sophistication of the services that the public demands, which would influence and likely couple with those established by governmental and private-sector, standards organizations, would likely determine the minimal standards that would ensure this quest to survive and be profitable. The issue of sophistication of expected health services would likely become increasingly important, as baby-boomers become seniors, hence the need to start to address these issues from now on. Healthcare providers, including hospitals, will not only stand a better chance to survive, but would likely be more profitable for example, as practitioners face fewer malpractice suits due to more widespread adherence to evidence-based practice, another often healthcare ICT-backed quality dimension. The combination of improved quality of care and its affordability would reduce the need for uncompensated care in countries such as the U.S., where it is a major healthcare costs driver. Attention to quality therefore could have far-reaching consequences capable of ensuring that we do not only meet the healthcare needs of the citizenry, but also that we curtail health spending, both critical achievements in health systems that would cater for an increasingly aging but equally increasingly discerning population.

An important contributor to healthcare consumers becoming more discerning is

access to more health and other relevant information. What does this tell us about a recent study that found that white, middle-aged Americans are not as healthy as their English counterparts are, and in both countries, that individuals with lower income and education levels have poorer health? The study published in the May 3, 2006, issue of the Journal of the American Medical Association[13], noted that among study participants, the healthiest Americans, persons in the highest income and education brackets, had diabetes and heart disease rates akin to those among the least healthy English individuals, those in the lowest income and education brackets. The National Institute on Aging (NIA), a component agency of the National Institutes of Health in the U.S. Department of Health and Human Services, and British government agencies funded the study. According to Dr. Richard J. Hodes, director of NIA, "This comparison raises some important questions about the relationship among health, education and income in both countries. As many nations try to address the challenges of population aging, it will be critical to know why these differences in health status appear." Richard M. Suzman, director of NIA's Behavioral and Social Research Program also noted, "This study challenges the theory that the greater heterogeneity of the U.S. population is the major reason the United States is behind other industrialized nations in some important health measures. By focusing on the comparable white populations, this study still finds the U.S. lagging". Americans also reported significantly higher levels of diabetes, twice as high, and heart diseases than did the English. Persons in the lowest income and education brackets in both countries had the highest rates of diabetes, high blood pressure, heart diseases, including heart attacks, strokes, and chronic lung disease, individuals in the highest income and education levels, the least. Cancer also showed this inverse relationship, the findings unexplained by differences in smoking, obesity and alcohol use between the countries. The researchers noted that the differences occurred despite higher U.S healthcare spending, similar smoking patterns, and identical life expectancies between the U.S and England. In seeking explanations for these puzzling findings, the researchers suggested some potential subjects of further research efforts, for example, the findings by earlier studies that different experiences with childhood disease could explain some of those observed in adult disease. Could social programs in the U.K help protect ill persons from loss of income and poverty, and could their lack in the U.S explain the greater link between health and wealth for its citizens that the study found, asked the researchers? The researchers also suggested that we would learn much extending the study to other countries with different health systems, for example, other European countries, and Canada, in particular examining the health of minorities, which would enable a comparison the effects of public funding of their health systems on health. There are indeed, likely to be many possible reasons for the observations emerging from this research, some of them operating individually, others in an elaborate interplay whose nature and intricacies would require a thorough analysis to tease out. Nonetheless, the findings indicate issues that need urgent attention in both countries, and in all other countries, developed and otherwise, now and in the years ahead, chief among which, disparities in healthcare services distribution, hence in healthcare delivery, but also important, the pervasive and chronic information asymmetry in the health systems of these countries. The findings also confirm a common knowledge that the relationship between health spending and the quality of healthcare delivery is not always a direct one, and is often in fact an inverse relationship. So, then why should we not seek ways to reduce spending while simultaneously providing high quality care, dual objects that healthcare ICT could help us achieve? Could the widespread diffusion of healthcare ICT help make healthcare ICT more affordable, hence more accessible even for the lowest income groups in privately funded health systems too? Could healthcare ICT, by helping to rectify the information asymmetry mentioned earlier also assist in providing individuals with the lowest education relevant health information that could improve their knowledge of health issues and make better able to embrace disease prevention and health promotion measures? Would such knowledge also make them more discerning regarding the choices of healthcare providers and other important decisions that they make regarding their health, which could lower the prevalence rates of diseases among them? Indeed, one of the problems that the disclosure of the entire costs of procedures that President Bush proposed, mentioned earlier, would solve, in this case regarding pricing, is the pervasive information asymmetry that continues to plague the health industry. This is why the disclosures should be all embracing, so that we do not have a partial solution to the information asymmetry in this domain. In other words, healthcare consumers should also have information on their out-of-pocket costs, and variations in prices, and why, for examples. A recent RAND California individual insurance market study shed some light on the complex relationships between pricing, information asymmetry, and healthcare delivery coverage, and indeed, quality. The California HealthCare Foundation funded the research, whose results the authors argued are likely applicable to other states. The study essentially concluded that slashing premiums did not enlarge coverage significantly in individual markets, and warned of the possibilities of adverse results high-deductible plans might engender. Published in a Health Affairs Web Exclusive on May 02, 2006, the researchers noted that a 20% premium subsidy would only result in a 5-11% increase in subscriber rate in the individual market and a 1-3% fall in the number of uninsured persons, coming from 1-2% rise in potential insurance buyers, and about 15% coverage dropout by fewer current enrollees. The study indicated that price breaks could help, but only minimally to increase coverage. Should we therefore not be looking into additional measures to increase coverage in our bid to rectify the disparities in healthcare delivery? Should this not be priority considering that these disparities could potentially increase the prevalence rates of diseases among the affected population, the cumulative effect of which would be an increase in healthcare spending, and a fall in the quality of overall health services as funds required to improve quality become scarcer? This report also noted that price subsidies could help promote whole family and continuity of coverage, but also not so efficiently since many who receive the subsidies would likely already have such coverage, price break regardless. Contrary to some people's apprehension, premium subsidies in the individual market would unlikely create chaos in the group market, as even a 20% subsidy has only a less than 0.05% reduction rate in worker participation in their own plan. The authors' answer to the question we posed earlier about increasing health coverage supports our earlier contention about the adverse consequences on health coverage and healthcare delivery quality of information asymmetry. Indeed, the authors of this report suggested that tackling non-price barriers, in particular, the difficulty in accessing information, might increase individual market participation as much, if not more than price subsidies. In other words, it is crucial that we provide healthcare consumers more information. According to the authors, purchase rates would increase by 9%, the same effect as a 20% subsidy if "one could reduce the perceived costs of search from the mean to the lowest twenty-fifth percentile of perceived information search costs." Further, reducing the average cost of information search to the level of the lowest tent h percentile would boost participation by 30%. There is no doubt about the increasing importance of the individual market in countries such as the U.S., where far from being interim measures to plug holes in group coverage, people, particularly the older consumers, take such coverage for the long haul, roughly 60% for over one year, and 30%, over three. Should we therefore not be taking such simple measures based on the targeted health information-dissemination principle, to provide the health consumer with the information required to expand this market, hence health services provision? The need for such information, for example, which broadens the scope of health consumers in making choices about actuarial products' value, hence acquisition, also was one of the observations the authors made. Roughly, 25% of individuals in 2002 that purchased individual products signed up in plans paying about 95% of total spending for a standardized population, about 25%, for plans covering less than 67%, which suggests variations in preferences, purchasers seemingly deriving value from the wider scope that individual relative to group markets offer. Would the health consumer provided more relevant information not have even better understanding of the operations of the markets, hence be better able to make the most rational choices based on his/her preferences? Would such choices not be crucial in cushioning the effects of or even eliminating adverse selection considering the concern of some "that the very diversity of products that insurers offer is an attempt to separate risks and charge them different prices?" Some studies have shown that there is substantial risk pooling in the individual market with high risks clients' premiums not fully reflective of such increased risks, which this study also confirmed. Furthermore, and according to the researchers, because the federal authorities, via Health Insurance Portability and Accountability Act (HIPAA) require "guaranteed renewal" those who enroll and become sick cannot be excluded from the pool, and in practice they are not placed in a new underwriting class". Should we therefore not continue to make information available that would enable more healthcare consumers to embrace the individual market since it seems to eliminate adverse selection? Alternatively, would the risk pooling and guaranteed renewal eventually result in "virtual" information asymmetry, hence proxy adverse selection with premiums going up? Furthermore, some argue, underwriting in this market shuts out some high-risk consumers in the first place, essentially placing persons that acquire coverage in better health than those uninsured, besides the suggestion of this study of the ease attracting healthy than high-risk subscribers to high-deductible plans. As the authors noted, "Currently, preferred provider organization (PPO) products with high cost sharing are primarily subscribed to by those in good health, and larger premium reductions are needed to induce subscribers in poor health to switch to high-deductible plans." This suggests the potential for advantageous rather than adverse selection in consumer-driven health plans because the insured are less at risk. It seems therefore that we need to be looking in both directions in establishing measures that would prevent both adverse and advantageous selections, hence, the edifice of the consumer-driven health model, crumbling. There is no doubt that rectifying the information asymmetry pertaining to the health industry is one such measure. Because we cannot afford to place the survival of insurance firms in jeopardy, we must also rectify the information asymmetry that pertains to the insurance industry. Adverse selection does not work for this industry as well. By pricing out low risk clients, the insurance firms risk non-profitability hence compromised competitiveness, and perhaps even extinction. Let us address this issue briefly. It might seem on first inspection that the industry already has all the information that it needs, but this is not necessarily the case, considering the pace of the growth of medical knowledge, and of information on both existing and emerging diseases. The elucidation of the genome for example continues apace, new information on the genetic origins of diseases, and the interaction of genes and the environment in the development of diseases surfacing incrementally. Such developments create the need for insurance firms to keep abreast of developments in the health industry, including knowledge of emerging diseases, and their treatments. This creates another dimension for the principle of targeted health information mentioned earlier. Should the need for such targeted information by the insurance industry trigger interest by knowledge management firms and information providers to provide such services and meet those needs, and would the insurance industry fully updated about medical knowledge not perform better in rational pricing and underwriting? Does this not imply that the industry also needs to embrace and implement healthcare ICT, for example, sophisticated data management systems and data mining technologies? Should our efforts at promoting healthcare ICT diffusion therefore not cut across industries, and healthcare stakeholders? With regard the information asymmetry, that hampers decision-making among healthcare consumers, would such information for example not prevent ex-ante moral hazard, coupled for example, with discounts if consumers did not engage in or quit adverse lifestyles, in the latter case, some form of positive reinforcement? Would this not ultimately lower premiums and make coverage more affordable, hence more widespread? Would such widespread coverage not improve the overall health of the populace, and with more consumers exercising their choice of providers, also the quality of service delivery? Would such information provision also not help reduce the prospects of ex-post moral hazard, for examples, the wastage, and the overuse of services that might result from our efforts to lower premiums, which could drive insurers out of business and further increase healthcare spending by government? Of course, some would argue that it is one thing for healthcare consumers to have information, and quite another for them to imbibe, and actualize its contents. We may need to come up with effective ways to ensure the attitudinal changes necessary for whatever measures we take to make increased health coverage work. One way to achieve this goal again is to implement the principles of targeted health information. Some might say "legislating health" is a better option, but this is disregarding the very essence of humankind, which is its rational nature, besides not acknowledging that of legislating, which is coercion. Just as consumers have the choice to embrace or jettison information, many might choose to break the law. This is not to say that legislation is not necessary regarding certain health issues, but would persuasion not work better in many instances, especially backed by "loss" of the sorts of positive reinforcement mentioned earlier. Would the prospects of such loss not encourage the financially challenged to imbibe targeted health information for example on healthy lifestyles, particularly as the report in *Health Affairs* mentioned earlier indicates that providing consumers with information is even more efficient than subsidy in increasing coverage? Substance dependence for example is a behavioral pattern but with biological roots, and which creating the impression that its perpetuation albeit circumscribed has no potentially adverse consequences for the person involved, his/her family, and society, belies. In other words, would fiat, or a thorough understanding of the diathesis, the individuals have coupled with whatever environmental concomitants confound it, likelier extinguish it? If the latter, should our approaches not therefore involve biological and environmental manipulation? Would establishing services along these lines, which would clearly involve significant information exchange, hence heavy healthcare ICT input, for example, regarding targeted, analyzed, and contextualized health information at teenagers that could discourage initiating illicit substance use, reckless sexual behaviors, and other high-risk activities, not help? Would such services not readily identify those teenagers with diathesis that warrant further, possibly biological treatment approaches, both efforts, overall reducing the rate of teenagers using illicit substances and engaging in other high risk behaviors? What would society be saving in human and material terms rather than adopting a somewhat naïve no-danger-in-circumscribed-use approach to this problem? Put differently, what would such latitude do to help individuals, with heavy genetic loading for substance dependence? Indeed, how would it, considering the domino effect of the use of illicit substances, help to prevent even the individual without such diathesis spiraling down the dependence abyss? Do the various adverse effects of alcohol and cigarette consumption we see around us not tell this story? Could any society afford to nurture a generation of youths dependent on illicit substances not addressing the issue of substance use, before it realizes the damage to the future of its health and social security services, and would the seniors have to fund health and social security services for examples under these circumstances? Should efforts to tackle substance use/dependence not start at its core?

Finding solutions to the health problems of our youths makes intuitive sense, not

only regarding the future of society, but also in looking ahead at caring for our seniors, who there are indications already that we are neglecting. A joint report by three public sector watchdogs in the U.K for example recently noted that the National Health Service (NHS) and care services treated seniors with a lack of dignity and respect, worsened by lack of consultation, according to the Audit Commission, Healthcare Commission, and Commission for Social Care Inspection[14]. The report evaluated the government's progress halfway through its 10-year plan to improve services for the over 50s. According to David Behan, chief inspector of the Commission for Social Care Inspection," The evidence from this study is that older people are not involved in the design of services and, consequently, services are not tailored to their needs and aspirations" It is vital to understand and respond to the specific needs of older people." Could the need to tailor services to the needs of our seniors be better put? Even now, as Anna Walker, chief executive of the Healthcare Commission, observed " Older people are the biggest users of healthcare, occupying almost two thirds of our hospital beds, yet they continue to be a low priority in both the planning and development of our health service. " Would this not even be worse down the road when we would have even more seniors and demands for health and social services would be likely even higher? Should we not intensify efforts to seek alternative ways to provide healthcare services to the elderly outside the hospital, which if we did not would mean even higher hospitalizations rates and longer stays, which of course could only further increase health spending? Could we not in fact provide even more qualitative health services to our seniors at less expense, out side the hospitals, the latter considered apical centers reserved for specialized rather than routine health services? Do all these not speak to the need to develop and strengthen ambulatory and domiciliary services? What role could healthcare ICT play in this regard? The U.K report noted that none of the 10 communities across England, whose public services underwent scrutiny, achieved all the government-set milestones to enable them to meet NHS standards, tow key areas of concern, the planning of public transport and the low priority given to foot care services, singled out, both crucial to the success of ambulatory/domiciliary services. The report also noted that mental health care, where services deteriorated significantly for citizens older than 65 years. There was also mention of discrimination against the elderly in public and social services. These are issues of concern that may not necessarily apply just to the U.K. but also many other countries both in the developed and developing world, and require urgent efforts to address and remedy. A significant proportion of the population in many of these countries comprises seniors and many more would become seniors over the years. Indeed, about 25 million persons worldwide have dementia with estimates in another tow decades double this figure. Baby-boomers, who represent those persons born after WWI and the mid-sixties, some would say specifically between 1946 and 1964, will become seniors in 2011. By some estimates, this makes one in every three Canadian a baby-boomer for example. Besides the general need for more health services that old age brings, seniors also tend to have a preponderance of certain diseases in the developed countries, for example. One such disease is Alzheimer's disease, the most common form of dementia, which accounts for roughly 65% of all dementias in Canada. Alzheimer's disease is a progressive, degenerative brain disease, not a normal part of aging, with no known cure. An estimated almost 300,000 Canadians over 65 have the condition, which affects more women than men, and another almost 150,000 other dementias. With baby-boomers becoming seniors, they will also be in the age of increased risk for Alzheimer's disease (AD), and with an estimated 97,000 Canadians expected to develop dementia in 2006 alone, and close to 4 million, to have AD or some form of dementia in two decades, there is no doubt that health service provision needs urgent focus[15]. Canada spends an estimated $5.5 billion a year on individuals with AD and other dementias[16]. This figure would likely increase based on projected increases in the percentage of the population that would have these conditions. Should we indeed, not be planning regarding how best to provide qualitative health services to our seniors while simultaneously reducing costs? Consider the following reports of the benefits of telehealth. There has been much commendation of an inventive healthcare scheme by Medway Council and Medway NHS and Teaching Primary Care Trust regarding the excellent coordination of care delivery that telemedicine offers, which, including facilitating the treatment and monitoring of chronic conditions, such as heart disease, high blood pressure, and diabetes, has led to a 67% reduction in hospitalization rates. The pilot scheme, which had 31 participants not only improved the quality of life (QOL) of persons with such conditions, but also optimized resource utilization by freeing up precious NHS resources, saving 133 hospital days and 117 nursing hours, besides cost and time for GPs, and community nurses, among others. Patients are able to measure their own blood pressure, heart rate, temperature, even ECG, and other parameters, via a monitor, the values recorded, and transmitted over a phone line to a secure server, saved there, where doctors and other authorized healthcare professionals could access them electronically. The monitor is also able to send alert signals in case it detects abnormal values to trained operators who would then notify the patient's family or other doctor. Is this not the direction health services should be going if we were serious about providing qualitative health services at reduced costs, and should other countries not implement these and other technologies that would facilitate such ambulatory/home care? With the prospects of close to two-thirds of persons receiving telehealth services not requiring family doctors' visits in one year, patients actively involved in their treatment hence empowered, quality of life (QOL) improved, and patients receiving treatment in the comfort of their own homes, among loved ones, and with prompt access to expert opinion, should they not? Would these countries not be achieving the dual objectives of high quality service provision and curtailed healthcare spending? The U.K Government has set aside an £80m Preventative Technologies Grant (PTG) funding to develop long term sustainable service delivery improvements via basic support measures to preempt imminent or future crises, and sustain well being and avert the use of expensive care. Should other countries also not invest in this area, the specific goals set, which healthcare technologies, for example telehealth, could help them achieve. Should we not in fact be looking at initiating more programs for seniors that telehealth could help actualize? This brings to mind the crucial issue of wait times, one that looms larger than perhaps any other healthcare delivery issue in some developed countries does, which viewed against the background of the increasing need for health services for seniors for example, and its cost implications, suggests a need for reconciliation of policy initiatives to harmonize future health services orientation. In Canada, for example, there is an ever-increasing demand for services in the declared priority areas of cancer, heart, diagnostic imaging, joint replacements, and sight restoration, many of the health issues related to these areas, chronic and commoner among seniors, hence in keeping with the demographics of the country. In a recent Canadian Institute for Health Information (CIHI) report titled, *Waiting for Health Care in Canada: What We Know and What We Don't Know*, there was a cautious suggestion that even this high demand has not appreciably increased wait times. The report noted for examples, a 51% increase (by 22 000 cases) between 1998 2003 in the number of cardiac bypass surgeries, and angioplasties; a 30% increase (up 11 340) in knee, and hip replacements; and a 32% increase (62 000 cases) in cataract surgeries. Although being the first time compiling comprehensive wait time data in the country, and a valid reference point lacking, the Institute noted that it is impossible to conclude whether the situation is improving, even if it has clearly not worsened. There is no doubt that more widespread healthcare ICT implementation would help with more accurately measuring wait times as data are scattered all over the country, and among a legion of practitioners and healthcare institutions required for such accurate assessments. Since wait times measurement is an important quality indicator of access to care, it should strengthen our resolve to pursue this goal of interoperable healthcare ICT diffusion even more vigorously. It also signals the need to encourage healthcare providers to use these technologies, including to communicate, and to share important wait-times data. The report projected approximately 50% of all patients wait less than 30 days for non-emergency surgery, much longer for hip and knee replacements, typically 3 months, that about 10% of all patients wait at least 6 months for treatment, that queues to see a specialist are in general long. It also noted that for hip and knee replacement, often 30% of the overall wait time was for awaiting the initial orthopedic consultation. There is no doubt that efforts should continue to reduce wait times but could more intensive efforts toward the ambulatory/community/domiciliary triangle of healthcare delivery, including promoting the widespread implementation of the relevant healthcare technologies to facilitate the efficient and effective actualization of these initiatives not in fact make the need for efforts to reduce wait times redundant? By being able to perform most of the treatment and monitoring of the conditions now done in hospitals in these different settings, would there not be less pressure, and indeed, less need for hospital attendance, and stays? Considering that seniors are some of the heaviest users of hospitals and who the issues of wait times concern the most, would we not be improving the quality of care that they receive relieving them the agony of prolonged wait for treatment in hospitals providing them with the treatment in these different settings, and even more cost-effectively? Would we not in fact be achieving the dual objectives mentioned earlier by so doing and in the case of Canada for example, thereby keeping faith with the Canada Health Act?

Interestingly, the March 28, 2006 Web Exclusive edition of *Health Affairs* published a

U.S. study that showed essentially that population aging plays a minor role in the growing demand for hospital services, essentially dispelling the widely held notion that aging baby boomers justify rapid expansion in hospital services, including the construction new hospitals[17]. Researchers at the Center for Studying Health System Change (HSC) apparently disagreed with this premise their study indicating that population aging will increase use of inpatient services between 2005 and 2015, by just 0.74% per year, 7.6% over the entire decade, compared with an estimated overall

64.8% rise in inpatient services utilization during the same period. The researchers noted the more significant roles that local population trends and medical technology advances would play in forecasting community needs for additional inpatient hospital capacity than population aging, which underscores the overarching theme of our discussion in this paper. This is that the pursuit of quality as a goal in itself and as a necessary component of our quest to deliver excellent health services to the populace and to reduce costs must start with the people themselves, with understanding and working towards delivering their expectations, which of course would reflect their needs. We have also stressed the need for formal metrics to measure quality based additionally on a thorough analysis of prevailing health and disease outcome indicators, demographics, and other measures crucial to accomplishing the service planning and resource utilization from which future qualitative services would emerge. The perpetuation of this quality determination, evaluation, and re-determination is the key quality cycle that any health system needs to meet the dual objectives mentioned earlier. The study calls for caution, no doubt, on the part of hospital CEOs who might be planning on extensive expansion projects because based on the idea that an aging population will result in increased demand for inpatient care. On the contrary, the direction of health services will be toward the less expensive, yet effective, and qualitative ambulatory/ domiciliary /community approaches to healthcare delivery, not least because, and as our discussion thus far shows, it presents us with excellent opportunities to achieve the dual goals mentioned above. The study projected the average age of the U.S population between 2005 and

2015 to increase only from 36.5 to 37.9 years, or an average annual increase of 0.37 percent. It also did not say that aging would not play any role, but in fact, that it would play a bigger role in increased inpatient utilization between 2005 and 2015 than in the previous decade the overall effect is just going to be relatively small, which is in keeping with the shift in the direction of healthcare delivery mentioned earlier. Indeed, the study, titled, "The Effect of Population Aging on Future Hospital Demand," also noted that the effects of aging vary widely across diseases treated in an inpatient setting, high for certain heart and orthopedic diseases, stable or falling some obstetric-related and mental illnesses. This again, underlines, the importance of analyzing, as we earlier discussed, the data fed into the quality metrics mentioned above, in not only evaluating the quality, but in re-determining future quality goals, and the actions that stream from them. The study also examined the comparative roles of aging versus medical technology. They used inpatient utilization rates for two cardiac procedures: coronary artery bypass graft (CABG) surgery and percutaneous transluminal coronary angioplasty (PTCA) to make this comparison, and found that the use of each between 1993 and 2002 had only age patterns changed, would have risen 0.6% yearly. Rather they found that 83.4% more persons had PCTA during an inpatient stay, or 7% per annum, during the period, 1.4%, or 0.2% more per annum for CABG surgery. These findings point to the fact that medical technologies would likely have a greater effect on hospital utilization, hence costs, than aging, or would it? The question is who are the people undergoing these procedures? Are they the older individuals in society, and if so, does that not make the effects of the medical technologies, proxy? Could we, by making it unnecessary not to or at least reducing the need to have these and other hospital-based procedures in fact reduce the rates of hospitalizations among these individuals? Would this likely happen considering as the authors of the study also noted that "Although aging will likely have an important impact on spending, its magnitude will be dwarfed by the impact of advances in technology and other factors that affect medical practice patterns" we could control these non-aging factors that influence paradigm shifts in medical practice? The specific findings of this study, for example, the rate of change in average age, may not apply directly to other countries, but it has broader implications for the likely changes that healthcare delivery would undergo in the near future, and the need to realign health policy formulation and initiatives in consonance with these likely changes. In Japan for example, renowned for its advanced robotics, a Japanese-led research team recently announced that it had made a seeing, hearing and smelling robot capable of carrying human beings aimed at helping care for the country's increasing seniors' population. The research institute, Riken, which developed the robot and receives robust Government funding, indicated that the 158-centimeter (five-foot) RI-MAN humanoid is currently capable of carrying a doll weighing 12 kilograms (26 pounds), and projects it would be able to carry one that weighs 70 kilograms within five years. According to Toshiharu Mukai, a research team member, "We're hoping that through future study it will eventually be able to care for elderly people or work in rehabilitation". The robot has a five millimeters (0.2 inches) soft silicone coat, sensors that show it a body's weight and position, weighs 100-kilogram (220-pound), and is able to tell between eight different kinds of smells, and from which direction a voice is coming, and is able to utilize powers of sight to trail a human face. The researchers envisage that the robot would be able to detect a human's health condition through his breath in the near future. Is Japan, which holds world records in longevity, even despite declining birth rates, not on the right track in preparing for expected major increase in needs for its seniors? Is that other countries worldwide would have to do the same moot, or imperative? With the constraint that our indubitably finite resources inevitably place on us, as is that the mandate of our responsibilities to humankind, the answer may not be far to seek.

References

1. Available at: http://www.kff.org/spotlight/longterm/index.cfm
Accessed on April 28, 2006

2. Available at: http://www.medicalnewstoday.com/medicalnews.php?newsid=42192
Accessed April 29, 2006

3. Available at: http://www.chcf.org/topics/chronicdisease/index.cfm?itemID=118083
Accessed on April 29, 2006

4. The Power of Prevention: Reducing the health and Economic Burden of Chronic Diseases 2003. Centers for Disease Control and Prevention. U.S. DHHS

5. Available at: http://www.ohqc.ca/en/yearlyreport.asp
Accessed on April 29, 2006

6. Available at: http://www.cbc.ca/news/adr/database/ Accessed on April 30, 2006

7. Available at: http://fermat.nap.edu/catalog/9738.html?onpi_newsdoc121499
Accessed on April 30, 2006

8. Available at: http://www.iom.edu/CMS/8089/5432.aspx Accessed on April 30, 2006

9. JAMA, December 14, 2005; 2858-2865

10. Available at: Article URL:

http://www.medicalnewstoday.com/medicalnews.php?newsid=42354 Accessed on April 30, 2006

11. Leatherman S, McCarthy D. *Quality of Health Care for Medicare Beneficiaries: A Chartbook*. The Commonwealth Fund, May 2005, Vol. 815. Available at: http://www.cmwf.org/publications/publications_show.htm?doc_id=275195 Accessed on April 30, 2006

12. Padmanabhan Ramnarayan, Graham C Roberts, Michael Coren, Vasantha Nanduri, Amanda Tomlinson, Paul M Taylor, Jeremy C Wyatt and Joseph F Britto, Assessment of the potential impact of a reminder system on the reduction of diagnostic errors: a quasi-experimental study. BMC Medical Informatics and Decision Making 2006, (in press) Available at: http://www.biomedcentral.com/bmcmedinformdecismak/ Accessed on May 01, 2006

13. Banks, J, Marmot, M, Oldfield, Z, and James P. Smith, Disease and Disadvantage in the United States and in England, Journal of the American Medical Association (JAMA) May 3, 2006. Vol. 295, No. 16

14. Available at: http://news.bbc.co.uk/go/pr/fr/-/2/hi/health/4848646.stm Accessed on May 04, 2006

15. Ostbye T., Crosse E. Net economic costs of dementia in Canada. Can Med Assoc J 1994; 151 (10): 1457-64.

16. Hux M, et al. Relation between severity of Alzheimer's disease and costs of caring. Can Med Assoc J 1998: 159 (5): 457-465.

17. Available at: http://content.healthaffairs.org/cgi/content/abstract/hlthaff.25.w141 Accessed on May 04, 2006

ICT and Competition in the Health Industry

Many do not believe that the conditions required for competition in the health industry to thrive exist [1,2]. Therefore, they have misgivings about the chances of such novel market-based answers to costs inflation as consumer-driven healthcare working. Victor Fuchs[2], for example, in a 1988 article titled "The Competition Revolution in Health Care," published in *Health Affairs*, listed one of these conditions as the presence of large numbers of sellers and buyers, none of either domineering, to prevent excessive influence on market prices. Some contend that hospitals in particular, are merging under payer-pressure and rationalizing services to enhance their bargaining power for higher prices, just what some argue skew the market and make it less efficient. Many contend that insurers are indeed, also following suit, consolidating, these developments, despite the possibility of there still being a buyer/seller tug, no doubt raising questions on whether they constitute true competition, whither healthcare delivery under these circumstances, and in particular, if headed astray, what to do to steer it back on track? As we would argue in this discussion, for example, what role could the appropriate deployment of healthcare ICT play in not only fostering true competition in the health industry, but also in making competitive forces work for us in realizing our healthcare delivery goals in the near future? By helping shape competition in the health industry, could healthcare ICT facilitate the achievements of our objectives to deliver qualitative healthcare to our seniors now for example, and down the road, to the millions of baby-boomers-turned-seniors, and indeed, to other members of society, cost-effectively? The U.S. spends up to $6,400 per capita on health, and Ford Motor Co. and the United Auto Workers are in a health care cost-cutting deal that will shear $850 million off Ford's annual health care costs and $5 billion off its long-term retiree health care liability, a deal that the former insists it needs to regain financial health. Millions in the U.S. are unable to afford health coverage, and healthcare costs are still soaring in, but this is not peculiar to the country. In Canada, projected health spending for 2005 according to data that the Canadian Institute for Health Information (CIHI) released on December 07, 2005, was $142 billion, about 10.4% of the country's GDP (10.1% in 2004), $114.0 billion in 2002. Forecasts for total health expenditures for 2003 and 2004 were $123.0 billion and $130.3 billion, an increase of 7.9% and 5.9%, respectively. Overall increase in health spending over 2004, was 7.7%, and adjusted for inflation rate, 5.5%. For 2005, CIHI projected the country's per capita to be up to $4,411, an increase of 6.9% over 2004. With over a third of the country's population expected to be over 55 years in a decade and a half, health expenditures as a proportion of the provincial and territorial government revenues expected to be over 40% [3], should there not be concerns over the future of its healthcare? In particular, with its population aging, and public revenues likely to reduce progressively for a number of reasons, including those related to demographic changes, do these concerns not in fact call for urgent actions to preempt their possible untoward outcomes? The picture of healthcare in most other developed countries is not much different from those of Canada, and the U.S., in terms of increasing healthcare costs, which the demographic changes occurring in these countries also threaten to escalate. Health spending is increasing at all payer levels irrespective of the funding and architecture of the health system, these payers taking action someway or another. With the proposed Ford/UAW deal mentioned earlier, for example, Ford hourly retirees would pay deductibles, premiums, and co-payments for the first time, up to $370 and $752 yearly for individuals and families, respectively, figures that could increase in the next few years depending on how much of two new trust funds would go into reducing payments. Further, active hourly workers will have to contribute portions of future pay increases to the trust funds, according to the deal, which Ford indicates will add $108 million to its fund by 2011. Total health expenditure per capita, that is, the per capita amount of the sum of Public Health Expenditure (PHE) and Private Expenditure on Health (PvtHE) for the U.K in 2002 was $2,160, the country's t otal expenditure on health as percentage of GDP was 7.7% in 2002, from 6.8% in 2000. NHS spending was about £67.4bn ($125.5 billion) in 2004-2005, and is increasing. Indeed, before the 2002 Spending Review the U.K Government asked Derek Wanless to evaluate "the financial and other resources required to (ensure) that the NHS can provide a publicly funded, comprehensive, high quality service on the basis of clinical need and not ability to pay". The review concluded that the UK should devote a considerably larger share of its national income to health care over the next two decades in order to catch up with the best-developed countries in half that time, and sustain this progress in the next half. It also noted that the success or otherwise of these efforts would depend principally on how effectively the health service employs its resources. This review examined three scenarios, one of them, a "fully engaged" scenario in which the public is highly engaged in health, life expectancy is longer than current forecasts, health status remarkably improves, resource use is more efficient, and health service responsive, and healthcare ICT diffusion more widespread. It is interesting to note that this is akin to our suggestion earlier that resource utilization is a major cost driver, and healthcare ICT properly deployed could reduce these costs yet ensure qualitative healthcare delivery. Indeed, the review went so far as to affirm that the fully engaged scenario was the least expensive scenario and that would deliver best health outcomes, and that in absolute expenditure terms embracing the best scenario could save as much as £30 billion by 2022/23, or half of current NHS expenditure, vis-à-vis, the worst. Mr. Wanless in April 2003, at the behest of the U.K Government provided an update of the challenges in implementing the fully engaged scenario set out in his report on long-term health trends, focused especially on cross-departmental work on preventative health measures and health inequalities. He published his final report

"Securing Good Health for the Whole Population", on February 25, 2004. Canada s increasing healthcare costs, an 11% more spending on prescription and non-prescribed medication, significantly higher than any other health spending, including on hospital services and doctors remuneration, much of its cause, understandably a cause for concern among policy makers, even the populace. Most of the prescriptions no doubt are for older Canadians, and those with chronic conditions. Is it therefore any wonder that the country is refocusing on healthcare issues relating to seniors, considering the demographic changes it is undergoing, its population becoming increasingly older? CIHI for example, on March 22, 2006, released information on continuing care, about which information was hitherto relatively scarce, titled Facility-Based Continuing Care in Canada, 2004 2005. The report, which provides information on continuing care facilities, hospital-based and nursing homes for examples, and their patients made a number of interesting observations, including that one in five continuing care patients cared for in Ontario hospitals is under the age of 65 years. By revealing the characteristics of continuing care patients, their needs, and how the health system is responding to them, the report creates a better understanding of the ability of continuing care facilities to meet the goal of care, which may not be curative, but to enable their clients to stay as healthy as possible, for as long as possible. It also facilitates policy formulation, resource planning, and allocation to rectify noted defects, and to monitor the quality of care and to improve service delivery. The report is CIHI s first on the subject, and utilizes data from hospital-based and nursing homes facilities in Ontario and Nova Scotia, with other provinces and territories, starting with Alberta, British Columbia, Manitoba, Saskatchewan, and the Yukon Territory, expected to begin submitting continuing care data to CIHI between 2006 and 2008. Pain, with 47 of clients experiencing unrelieved pain, and 10%, severe daily pain, is a key complaint among many hospital-based continuing care patients, most of who, admitted from an acute care hospital bed, are not all elderly, as many as one in five (18%), less than 65 years old in 2004/2005. The report also showed that 22% were dependent completely on others for the basic activities of daily living (ADL), 82% had multifarious and unstable health conditions. Twenty four per cent of clients showed evidence of depression, 59% of those admitted for over 15 weeks had little, or no social interest, which likely reflect the serious health conditions or disabilities many have, compared to nursing home residents, who were more socially engaged, and over half of who were 85 years or older. The 2004/05 Nova Scotia nursing-homes data show that half of the clients were from home, were on average, eight years older, were more likely to be pain-free, and their health more stable, and were less dependent for their ADL than their counterparts in hospital-based care, were, 33% discharged to hospital and 12% died in the facility. These findings, if applicable to the rest of the country raise many important issues regarding healthcare provision, in particular for seniors, and those with chronic diseases, many of who also happen to be older individuals. What does the fact that most of the clients in hospital-based facilities were from the hospital, whereas most of those in nursing homes were from home, the former, more physically unhealthy, and that a third of nursing home clients ended up in hospitals imply regarding the notion that an aging population such as in Canada would overwhelm the health services? These issues are important because an aging population per se will not increase healthcare costss, but the prevalence patterns of diseases, and nature and extent of health services that they need could. To be sure, healthcare costs will likely increase as the population ages, albeit slowly buffered by the economy, just 1% annually in total healthcare costs for the entire country, some contend6 but could increase steeply and substantially except other age groups service utilization remains stable. In the mid-1960s, the young and middle aged were responsible for roughly 70% of healthcare costs in British Columbia, about 33% to seniors, the situation reversed by the mid-1990s, even factoring in the hospital closures of the time. This latter is a key observation regarding our thesis in this discussion that healthcare ICT deployed appropriately, for example, in the efficient and effective operations of ambulatory/community/domiciliary care, could negate the increasing healthcare costs seniors incur, and the role competition, even in a publicly funded health system could play in this regard. Consider the case of Quebec, where the seniors' population in the decade starting in the early 1980s increased from 8.9% to 11.2%, the costs of physician services, twice as much as before. Increased doctors' remuneration, and in the numbers of older people, were partly responsible, but it was mostly due to the increased numbers of visits to the doctor[7]. This clearly demonstrates the importance of service utilization as a healthcare cost driver, but the question remains why seniors are utilizing services more than ever before. Could it be due to increasing longevity causing more ill health, or changing disease patterns that necessitate more contact with healthcare providers, or could the treatment of even these new diseases be different, and more cost-effective? Alternatively, are seniors not necessarily more ill, but healthy seniors seeing their doctors even more than unhealthy ones, in a seeming over-use of third-payer coverage, the so-called, "moral hazard?" Would such unnecessary consultations in particular with specialists, most of who are in hospitals not skyrocket costs, particularly in health systems that use capitation and/or fee-for-service remuneration systems for doctors? Are some seniors receiving treatments and procedures that have little benefits in improving their living standards, yet driving healthcare costs up? How important are ethico-moral issues such as "Do not resuscitate" (DNR) orders, and equitability in matters of healthcare costs? Are doctors not already playing a role, albeit passively in DNR compliance? Are they also going to be playing a more active role in assisting patients to die, and what would be the ethical and costs implications of this increased participation? Are these issues likely to feature more prominently in healthcare in the years ahead?

Indeed, they are already. Oregon, in the U.S., and the Netherlands, for examples

already have laws permitting doctor assisted dying, and there is a controversial debate going on in the British House of Lords regarding amending the laws to enable doctors assist the terminally ill to die. Will these debates surface at some point in other legislative Houses in the developed world, including for examples, Canada, and Australia, down the road? How would such laws if enacted affect our conceptualizations of healthcare delivery to seniors, and with the population in many countries aging, would these issues result in major policy and institutional changes in how each country funds and delivers healthcare? Lord Joffe's Bill would apply to those in England and Wales expected to die within six months and suffering agonizingly, but still able to make decisions. He told the peers in the House of Lord's debate on May 12, 2006, that patients should not have to endure such pain "for the good of society as a whole". However, not all the Lords agreed, with Lord Carlile insisting that the bill would result in doctors giving lethal drugs, and may lead to voluntary euthanasia, when the doctor actually helps the patient die. The Bill advises that upon signing a legal declaration of their intention to die, patients could receive a prescription of a lethal dose of medication that they could take to end their lives. Some contend that the Bill would unlikely become law but a YouGov survey of 1,770 people for Dignity in Dying (formerly the Voluntary Euthanasia Society) found 76% were in favor of assisted dying provided there were safeguards in place. The controversy over the Bill underlines the deep split between those in favor of the right to die and those who prefer better palliative care. There is no doubt that some patients suffer unbearably, sometimes for years, from terminal illness the agony, their families inexorably share. This is apart from the other costs, for example, financial, of treating them, which oftentimes their families also share. In many cases, even in the U.K, where palliative care is a medical specialty, it is difficult to meet the needs of these patients, who often express the wish to die, and free themselves and their families of suffering and pain. The 2004/05 Nova Scotia nursing-homes data mentioned earlier showed 33% of the patients, discharged to hospital. Should the province, for example, enact laws to allow those of these individuals, mostly seniors, who wish to die because of terminal illness in the nursing home, to do so? Could the province save substantially in hospital costs doing so? Should other Canadian provinces and territories enact such laws, too? Some would answer in the affirmative, and could argue that patients still able to take such decisions for themselves, should be able to do so, after the law allows relatives to take DNR decisions for patients unable to take such decisions themselves. With the U.K Bill having to pass through the Commons even if passed by the peers, it has major obstacles in the way, and obstacles there are. Archbishop of Canterbury Dr Rowan Williams is a key opponent of the bill, for example. U.K's Cardinal Murphy O'Connor cautioned that the Bill could result in pressure on vulnerable persons to end their own lives. A Royal College of Physicians poll showed that 73% did not support changing the present law. The Royal College of GPs has also changed its earlier neutral stance after members opposed the proposed law. These issues are doubtless, among those that would be the subject of debates in many countries, particularly as many more people live longer, and resources become even scarcer. If the goal of the Bill were to prevent needless suffering, could we not decompose the issue to explore whatever options we have hence perhaps assuage both parties on the opposite sides of the debate? Could we not consider suffering as physical or psychological as a starting point, for example? Let us assume that physical suffering is pain and loss of mobility, and discomfort due to difficulty eating or breathing, for examples, and psychological suffering, depression, and demoralization, and other what we could call psychic distress. Could we not seek better ways to ease these sufferings, and would doing so not ease those of their families too, some of who might be distressed, even if only psychologically seeing their relative go through such sufferings? Consider the findings in the following recent study, which indicates that we could improve the quality of care that patients with Alzheimer s disease receive. We are likely to care for most of these seniors with dementia increasingly in primary care setting, by primary care physicians. However, these setting confront major obstacles to achieving the goal of providing the seniors with qualitative care. A recent research study published in the May 10, 2006 issue of the Journal of the American Medical Association (JAMA) tested the effectiveness of a collaborative care model to improve the quality of care for patients with Alzheimer disease (AD). The study was a controlled clinical trial of 153 older adults with AD and their caregivers, who doctors randomized to receive collaborative care management (n = 84) or augmented usual care (n = 69) at primary care practices at 2 US university-linked health care systems between January 2002 and August 2004. Eligible patients met AD diagnostic criteria and had a self-identified caregiver. Intervention patients received a year care management that an interdisciplinary team provided. The team leader was an advanced practice nurse that worked with the patient s family caregiver and incorporated in primary care. The treatment approach involved the use of standard protocols in treatment and to identify, track, and treat dementia's behavioral and psychological symptoms, nonpharmacologically, stressed, with neuropsychiatric Inventory (NPI) administered at baseline and at 6, 12, and 18 months to evaluate primary outcome. Secondary outcome measures were the Cornell Scale for Depression in Dementia (CSDD), cognition, activities of daily living, resource use, and caregiver's depression severity. The results showed that 89% of intervention patients triggered at least one protocol for behavioral and psychological symptoms of dementia, the mean, four per patient from 8 possible protocols. Intervention patients received cholinesterase inhibitors and antidepressants, more, and had significantly fewer dementia's behavioral and psychological symptoms, measured by the total NPI score at 12 and 18 months. Their caregivers also reported significant improvements in distress, measured by the caregiver NPI at 12 and 18 months, and in depression, measured by the Patient Health Questionnaire-9. The CSDD, cognition, activities of daily living (ADL) or on rates of hospitalization, nursing home placement, or death showed no group variations. The researchers concluded that collaborative care for AD treatment showed a significant improvement in the quality of care and in dementia's behavioral and psychological symptoms among primary care patients and their caregivers, improvements achieved without any notable need to increase the utilization of antipsychotics or sedative-hypnotics. Should we not be exploring such collaborative management approaches in terminal illnesses, considering their prospects in not only helping the patient but also their caregivers, and the opportunities to manage the seniors in the community, with the significant savings in health costs that would engender? Another approach to decomposing the matter is to determine the threshold of suffering. This might be easier to do with pain, for example, hence we could establish what level of pain would be unbearable, except that even cultural factors play a part in response to pain, some more stoic than others are, confronted with similar pain levels. It would likely be equally dicey to attempt to quantify other forms of suffering in order to determine whose pain to consider unbearable. Without such measurable parameters, the laws would likely lead to abuse, perhaps a burnt-out caregiver, a spouse, or child perhaps, pressuring the ill to die, some even to hasten the transition of property, a clearly plausible but gross unintended consequence of such a Bill. Yet another approach to decomposing the problem is to consider its origins, which could assist us in devising better approaches to management, for example, understanding the biological roots of the depression following stroke, and not simply attributing it to loss of mobility, and other functional losses, which could be involved, too, nonetheless. The treatment of the depression then would be multifaceted, employing both pharmacological and psychological treatment modalities, in other to obtain the best results. We also need to consider personality characteristics for examples, which could determine which patient adopts a fatalistic, and which, a positive approach to his/her condition. In order to prevent the sort of abuse mentioned above, we need to examine the matter closely along these and other dimensions. This would involve a variety of processes, which healthcare ICT could help facilitate, for example, helping to elucidate the biological, psychosocial, and other issues that we could exploit in both understanding the individual and his/her needs better, and in developing appropriate management approaches in order to make the person s final days less distressing. Because these end-of-life issues would involve mostly seniors, they constitute aspects of their health that should not only be of legitimate concern, but that should warrant urgent attention, in order to prepare for the surge in the numbers of seniors, not only when baby-boomers become seniors, but also in the years ahead, long after that. Because we are likely to continue to see more seniors than ever before in the history of humankind, and because of such issues as discussed above, with society wary of being seen to condone " suicide" , why could some not argue that we should not stop the young man tired of living from declaring unbearable psychic pain, hence seek assisted dying? Why, they might insist should the young man want to have to saddle himself with the tax burden to fund healthcare for an increasing number of seniors for example? Besides, would it feel right for to-be seniors, for example, baby-boomers to contemplate someone pressuring them to death in their old age, because of some "unbearable" distress? Are these situations not going to make competition, which we could trace to the root of such pressure somewhat Hobbessian? Indeed, competition, at least in the present age should not, and need not be. In fact, competition ultimately serves the common, rather than the individual goal, the Leviathan, rather than being the umpire, the facilitator. In other words, the operations of competitive forces could make the debate on the U.K Bill essentially redundant. In order to appreciate why this is so, we need again to decompose competition, into two broad subsystems, each further into two dimensions, the first subsystem, its elements, the second, its consequences. Living beings and transactions are its elements, the latter, essentially information communication, the cobblestone, as one cannot sell even the greatest mansion, or want to buy it without such information passed from buyer to seller or vice versa. Its consequences are pecuniary/material and/or psychological/physiological fulfillment. These subsystems interact reciprocally to work for, and not against survival, and until our psycho-physiological systems, which even in the face of extreme hazards stubbornly attempt to compensate and keep working, become moribund and shutdown, continue to work for survival. It is admissibly complicated to conceptualize a dying individual as engaged in competition, but that is what survival is all about, that conceptualization easier if one considered the subsystems in universal terms. Thus gaseous exchange between our lungs and blood stream, or the struggle for calcium between the latter and our bones, for examples are transactions between two organ systems, or living beings. Bodily transactions even involve lending and borrowing, as in "oxygen debt" or excess post-exercise oxygen consumption, when because our muscles could not obtain enough oxygen as during rigorous exercises, they obtain energy anerobically, and must pay the oxygen back after the exercise, which is why we continue to breathe heavily to take in as much oxygen as possible. If therefore, we subscribe to the fact that survival, and not death is our natural state, terminating life even when terminal, rather than letting it expire on its own would be unnatural. Needless, to say, there have been individuals with grave illnesses, both physical and psychological, that have done great things for humanity despite these illnesses. Even taking a DNR decision for another who lacks the competence to do so should not be whimsical. Further, rather than give their patients some pill to take in order to die, doctors, who swore to the Hippocratic Oath to do no harm, should rather seek ways to enhance the competitive processes of living, or at the very worst, let them take their natural turns. Enhancing these processes involve facilitating the subsystems of the competitive processes of living, which should be all-inclusive, involving primary, secondary, and tertiary prevention, all of which the appropriate deployment of healthcare ICT could help achieve. In the particular case of the terminally ill, for example, most of the process facilitation would be for tertiary prevention, which essentially is minimizing the sequelae of whatever diseases an individual has including the use of require rehabilitation, and/or palliative programs. Thus, we should implement and use the appropriate healthcare ICT for example for a terminally ill person who has a physical illness but is still in an outstanding mental frame that would enable him/her enjoy life with his/her spouse, children, grandchildren. His/her family members could still imbibe a few lessons from him/her, that could inspire great innovations by say a grandchild in future that would be of immense benefits to humankind. Some would argue that keeping terminally ill patients alive that could not benefit from medical care is not cost-effective, but would we rather wish all our seniors away? The fact is that most of us would eventually become seniors, with people living increasingly longer. Some living beings such as tortoises live for over two hundred years, and some human beings, well past a hundred years. Do these not tell us that we could one day discover the secret of longevity? Scientists are making great strides in understanding regeneration of our organ systems, and might soon be able to develop the drugs to enable such regeneration in all our organs. So, if old age is here to say, should we not be exploring ways to manage the health of our seniors more in a cost-effective, yet qualitative manner? A report in volume 25, no. 3 issue (May, 2006) of *Health Affairs*, for example noted that the U.S, had fewer practicing physicians, practicing nurses, and acute care bed days per capita than the median Organization for Economic Cooperation and Development (OECD) country. Yet, it spent more on health care per capita than the median OECD country that year, $5,635 per person or two-and-a-half times the $2,280 OECD countries average, 48% higher than Norway, the second-highest spender with per capita health spending at $3,807. The researchers also noted that the

U.S. spends more than other countries mainly because of higher prices for health care goods and services. Interestingly, the report also noted that the U.S. spent 43 cents per capita on health technology, less than one-tenth that by Australia, the second-lowest spender on health technology. According to the study, Canada and Germany spend $31.85, and $21.20 per person, respectively, on healthcare ICT, the researchers noting that the U.S. lags "at least a dozen years" behind other industrialized countries in electronic health records (EHR) adoption. Yet, again, the researchers noted that one proposal for both lowering health spending and improving quality is the adoption of health information technology (HIT), just what we have been saying about achieving the dual objectives of qualitative healthcare delivery yet reduced health spending in our discussion in this paper. By fostering competition, could the widespread diffusion of healthcare ICT not help reduce the high prices of healthcare goods and services in the U.S that this study found? Would this not help reduce the country's soaring healthcare costs, eventually? In other words, even if some of the pecuniary benefits of healthcare ICT implementation are not immediately obvious, is it not worth the wait for them to eventually materialize considering that these technologies also help improve the quality of healthcare delivery, which effect are likelier to manifest in the short term? What role could healthcare ICT-backed preventive health programs play in reducing frivolous consultations, for examples, no doubt key healthcare costs drivers? How could competition help prevent such "moral hazard in a publicly funded health system such as in Canada? The U.K's health system is, as is Canada's, also essentially taxation-funded, and similarly facing potential fundamental changes, in particular regarding the nature and extent of free-market operations in the health system. Recent developments for example in the U.K have led to increased attention on improving efficiency, equity, and agility, in the NHS, the 2002, "Delivering the NHS Plan," whose purpose and vision, "is to give the people of Britain a health service fit for the 21st century:.. a health service designed around the patient, "one such development. Among its objectives is to offer patients increased choice of hospitals even if they do not have as much latitude regarding treatment. Thus, with effect from mid-2004, all patients waiting six months for surgery have the choice to obtain treatment from another hospital or provider within the country, and even overseas. On Thursday, June 09, 2005, the Supreme Court of Canada in *Chaoulli v. Quebec* ruled that the Quebec government could not prevent people from paying for private insurance for health-care procedures covered under Medicare. Four of the seven justices ruled that the provincial policy violated the Quebec charter. However, they split 3-3 on whether it did, the Canadian Charter of Rights and Freedoms, one judge abstained. This means that the ruling had no instantaneous effect on the Canadian health-care system as a whole, although some other provinces have signaled their intention to allow private healthcare, and private businesses have started companies offering private health services. Most countries are under relentless pressure due to rapidly increasing health expenditures despite dwindling resources, and worse still many not having much to show for the escalating health spending by way of qualitative healthcare delivery. Cost containment is thus one of the most viable options for these countries, which is triggering health organization and financing reforms, among others in many of these countries. Nonetheless, with extensive public borrowing no longer a viable economic policy in many countries, generating revenues to fund sustainable healthcare becomes a focus of consideration, hence the need for urgent revenue reforms. These considerations also bring those of competition to the fore regardless of whether the health system's funding model is public, private, or mixed.

Every country would like to provide its citizens the best health services, presumably. The problem is where to find the money to do so. Even in the developed world, resources are not limitless. Much is ongoing even in these countries to find reasons for increasing healthcare costs, which is a prerequisite to solving the problem. In the U.S for example, as we noted earlier, not only is its health spending significantly more than in other countries, including the developed ones, there are concerns that the value obtained from this spending is disproportionately smaller. Some have looked for answers to these disparities in the utilization of Intensive Care

Units (ICU) in the U.S. versus other countries such as the U.K., whose middle-aged citizens, a recent study published in the May 03, 2006 issue of the Journal of the American Medical Association are healthier than their U.S. counterparts. Research evidence suggests that ICU services in the U.S. account for a significant percentage of inpatient costs, the U.K., with significantly less number of ICU beds than the U.S.[8,9] There is no doubt that these differences would account for some of the differences in the health expenditures of these countries. There are of course significant differences in the population of both countries that could account for the disparities in the numbers of ICU beds, and indeed, the nature and extent of service utilization in both countries as well. The question is if both countries, and in particular the U.S. could not reduce the need for intensive care units by for example, reducing the need for surgeries; emergency and elective, accidents; and other reasons for the use of these services? Another question is if, indeed, their use would likely escalate in future, particularly because aging is now an integral part of our existence and, barring any catastrophe, we are unlikely to see fewer seniors in society than in generations past. It clearly makes intuitive sense to expect that the more seniors are in society, the higher would be health service utilization, but we should remember that the extent of use of such services as the ICU would also depend on other factors such as the degree of risk-taking by individuals, young and old. For examples, extreme sports, excessive drinking, and driving under the influence of alcohol, and drugs, among other accident-prone behaviors could increase sharply ER and possibly even ICU use, and hospitalization rates. Our efforts to reduce the use of such services must therefore cut across all age groups. Would efforts focused on preventing "moral hazard" help reduce the prevalence of risk-related accidents and injuries, for examples? Would this become a major issue in publicly funded health systems such as in Canada? There is no doubt that each person needs to be able to take some responsibility for his/her actions, if they could and should? In an article in the April 24, 2006 issue of *Maclean's,* on healthcare for patients with self-destructive vices, such as overeating, smoking, drinking or drugs, the magazine noted that some doctors in Canada are turning the patients away, or removing them from their waiting lists. According to the magazine, the doctors' argument included that it does not make sense to spend substantial amounts of money on treatments that are futile. Many would agree for example that it probably does not make sense to transplant livers to drinkers who would only start drinking all over again destroying the new organ, eventually. Just as they probably also would regarding treating a patient for chronic cough who would not quit smoking. Others would insist that the doctors were discriminating against these patients, and that this is in contravention to the Canada Health Act. The actions the doctors took have resulted in mixed results, in one instance, a tribunal dismissing a patient's complaints, in many cases, though, the patients quitting the habits, and remaining in treatment. These results point to one significant fact: the possibility of voluntary attitudinal change, after all the patients could have gone to other doctors since Medicare is essentially free, which counters any argument for coercion. Could we therefore, not develop contextualized programs, facilitated by the deployment of sophisticated healthcare ICT in achieving the same results, that is, attitudinal change, for example, regarding risk-taking, and other preventable causes of increased service utilization in ICUs, ERs, and hospitals, thus cutting down healthcare costs substantially? Could the ability of doctors to effect such attitudinal changes offer an approach for example in determining remuneration, as in pay-for-performance, or in determining incentives, or some form of reward? There is no doubt that surgery on chronic cigarette smokers, or very overweight or obese individuals carry substantial risks, regarding anesthesia for example, unrelated to the conditions for which they are receiving surgery. Nicotine for example compromises healing, failure rates for bone surgeries more than double among smokers. Would an orthopedic surgeon with a preponderance of patients that are chronic smokers, say, to who these patients flock, after rejection by other surgeons, not start to look like he/she is incompetent after some time? Could this picture, known to the public for example, via information on doctors as are in fact already starting to be available to the public on the Internet posted by an increasing number of health jurisdictions in the U.S, and Canada, for examples, not negatively influence patient enrollment with such practices? Now, even in publicly funded health system, could this not reduce the reimbursement that doctor receives from his/her employers, while increasing that by some other surgeon? Would the former surgeon not likely take measures to rectify this situation, for example, those that his colleagues took that resulted in attitudinal changes in their patients? In doing so, is this surgeon not making his/her practice more competitive? Would the cumulative effect of such competition not reduce the overall healthcare costs, while making the populace healthier by reducing the prevalence rates of preventable diseases? Would the process described above not even be faster were the doctors that institute programs to engineer such attitudinal changes rewarded in some way or another, besides the reward of seeing their patients get well faster, and take measures to prevent becoming ill in the future, and of course, their usual, if not increased remuneration? Our discussion so far therefore underscores the importance of competition in any health system, even in publicly funded ones and those with free universal health in achieving the dual objectives of delivering qualitative health services, while simultaneously reducing healthcare costs. The nature and intensity of the competition would vary depending on the country, its infrastructure, its institutions, its political and economic underpinnings, and its health funding structure, but it is nonetheless competition, and it is sine qua non to achieving the dual goals mentioned earlier. What is also crucial to how this competition plays out, hence to achieving these goals is the widespread implementation, and use of healthcare ICT. From the nature of the messages the doctor sends out to his/her patients, and the delivery medium, to measures, such as blood tests that the patients could perform at home, and transmitted automatically and wirelessly to the doctor's computers that could indicate compliance with behavior change, these technologies are offering today's healthcare provider opportunities for sophisticated value propositions. The variety of care provided to meet the determined needs of a healthcare provider's client base would increasingly be crucial to the practice's competitiveness, and in the end, survival, regardless of the health system's funding structure. With the increasing devolution of health services administration in many countries, including Canada, the dynamics of the relationships between payers and providers are going to be more complex over time, as patients become increasingly discerning, due for example to the likely evolution of competition among surgeons described above, and as the full ramifications of contemporary healthcare delivery saga unfold. We should of course be taking other measures in tandem with manipulating healthcare providers remuneration in order to trigger competition, as part of our overall efforts, for example, to rectify the information asymmetry that pervades the health sector, and indeed, related sectors, such as insurance. The process described above could be effective in reducing the effect of the anticipated increase in health service utilization among seniors in the years ahead, in terms of the economic burden of healthcare delivery, and that on the seniors and their families. However, we need to start now to examine our options in initiating this process, and it does not appear that we have done that thus far, at least sufficiently, to give the reassurance required to soothe the public s frail nerves, as the following story from *USA Today* shows. The paper on May 09, 2006 examined the challenges of rectifying the information asymmetry mentioned above, a crucial task were we to trigger the competitive processes mentioned above, successfully. According to the paper, although government and industry officials are encouraging Americans to shop better for healthcare, in order to boost competition in the health care marketplace and reduce healthcare costs, consumers lack ready access to reliable quality and pricing data that they need to compare health care services. The paper noted that health consumers could obtain quality information such as mortality and complication rat es, for some hospitals and procedures, but hardly for individual doctors. It further noted that because pricing data reflect the average charges that people pay rather than actual negotiated rates, consumers would not find them too helpful, if at all. These difficulties, among others, such as costly health care decisions often made by the ill, and often under emergency conditions, compromise the chances of the healthcare market operating efficiently, and effectively. Concerned that many doctors would not directly give a figure to the question on how much a service costs, and about the sometimes-wide variations in the prices of services in different states, or even parts of the same state, some employers and coalition of employers are seeking insurers willing to post actual price, and quality information for doctors and hospitals. This would no doubt facilitate price comparisons, and the paper profiled some insurers such as UnitedHeealthcare, Humana, Aetna, and HealthMarkets, giving such information, for example, via a network established for the coalition members. The efforts of these employers underscore the need for rectifying the information asymmetry referred to above, as a prerequisite for achieving the healthcare costs reduction that we hoped the healthcare consumer being able to choose healthcare providers, and the competition that this would engender, would bring. Indeed, the employers' efforts would likely pay off with many more insured workers armed with the information they need to negotiate pricing. This issue is the subject of a controversial bill currently tabled in the U.S. Senate. Sponsored by Sen. Mike Enzi, R-Wyo. the Bill, which the White House supports would enable businesses to join across state lines to purchase health insurance, with the polling expected to give them enough power to negotiate better coverage rates. This would enable small businesses to offer coverage to more workers, according to the Republicans. The Democrats however, contend that it would actually reduce health insurance for millions, in particular by preempting state requirements for coverage in some instances, for examples, for mammograms, or diabetes supplies, to which the Bill's sponsor responded that he would support some mandated coverage if a majority of the states requires it, a concession many believe could prevent a filibuster. There is no doubt that early detection and treatment of cancer could help reduce morbidity, and mortality, hence save costs, and not having cancer screenings, such as mammograms, cervical cancer screenings, and colorectal examinations, due to lack of coverage could result in the opposite effects, the idea behind state-mandated coverage. However, some contend that such mandates are actually driving up the costs of premiums, hence the numbers of the uninsured. Were this so, what would be the effect of even those that have coverage not undergoing screening either by choice, or because they are unaware of how and where to obtain these tests? Short of mandating individuals to have these tests, we need to come up with additional measures to persuade people that need them to take the tests. This underscores the need for targeted health information to such individuals.

Consider also the recent U.S Food and Drug Administration (FDA) release on

Tuesday 9, 2006 that there is no plausible scientific evidence that drinking green tea reduces the risk of heart disease, in rejecting a petition seeking to let tea labels make that claim, even after reviewing 105 articles and other publications submitted along with the petition. Some green tea companies claim that drinking at least five ounces of green tea a day may reduce the risk of heart disease, which the FDA has now refuted, and had actually also noted on June 30, 2005, that green tea likely does not reduce breast, prostate or any other type of cancer risk. Is this not important information that the many, and there must be millions of them around the world, who believe in the health benefits of the beverage need to know? There is no doubt that they could continue to drink the beverage but at least they know that they not doing so strictly because of its health benefits. Should the public also not know for example, that the FDA approved on May 11, 2006, a second medication to help smokers quit the habit, Pfizer's Varenicline, which research has shown helps one in five persons jettison the habit? Pfizer Inc. will be marketing the drug as Chantix, for twice-daily use. Varenicline reduces the enjoyment of smoking and the withdrawal symptoms that drives smokers to smoke repeatedly. There are already nicotine-substitution drugs on the market sold by prescription and over the counter (OTC) in a variety of forms such as patch, gum, patch, lozenge, nasal spray, even inhaler. Varenicline offers options to those that have tried the other drugs unsuccessfully. The FDA approved an antidepressant, bupropion, its anti-smoking brand called Zyban, as an anti-smoking drug. In studies conducted in Europe, and presented at the November 2005, conference of the American Heart Association, one year, abstinence rates were 22%, 16%, and 8%, for Varenicline, Zyban, and placebo, respectively, and after three months, 44% and 30% for the first two, respectively, the latter figures, according to Pfizer. Experts think that one should take it for much longer than three months, though, considering how hard it is to quit smoking. Varenicline attaches to the same brain receptors as nicotine does, and blocks the latter from releasing dopamine from the brain's pleasure centers, in addition to slowing dopamine's release, thereby reducing craving, in effect preventing the highs, and lows of cigarette smoking. With about 45 million Americans cigarette smokers, and smoking and related illnesses responsible for the deaths of almost half a million Americans every year, and a significant burden of illnesses in economic and human terms, there could be no gainsaying the benefits of such medications as Varenicline. There is also no doubt that we should intensify efforts to prevent people, particularly our young people from starting the habit in the first place. As Dr. Scott Gottlieb, the FDA's Deputy Commissioner for Medical, and Scientific Affairs noted, "Tobacco use, particularly cigarette smoking, is the single most preventable cause of death in the United States and is responsible for a growing list of cancers, as well as chronic diseases including those of the lung and heart". Should we not therefore make the information about this FDA approval widely available to those who need it, rather than expect them to search for it in the medical or other literature? The point here is that the public needs information, and there is no doubt about the immense role that healthcare ICT could play here, to assist it in understanding their health matters better. The availability of current and accurate information would also help the health consumer in taking decisions of the sort required to make any effort to improve the quality of healthcare delivery while at the same time saving health care costs work. The healthcare industry is undeniably information-intensive, compounded by the fact of the constant changes in a large part of this information based on progress in medical knowledge. In the first place, the health consumer needs information not just regarding diseases and other health issues including pricing of procedures, but also on doctors' profiles, hospital accreditation status, service offerings, and relating to accountability issues, among others. There is no doubt that it would be difficult for the average consumer to keep up with this information load. Should we therefore not make it possible for the consumer to receive those that he/she needs, contextualized, targeted, and delivered as frequently as practicable based on agreed contracts? It is important for us to appreciate this concept of targeted health information, as it is one of the most cost-effective ways to rectify the perennial information asymmetry hindering progress in the health industry. This information asymmetry also, in the main underlies the prohibitive costs of healthcare delivery, without much quality to show for it. Therefore, we need to intensify efforts to rectify the information asymmetry prevalent in the health industry, which developments in the industry are increasingly changing, indeed, urgently. Unlike only a year ago, as a Kaiser Family Foundation/Harvard/USA TODAY survey showed, relatively small numbers of consumers, only 11% of adult consumers negotiated with a healthcare provider for lower prices, many more would increasingly not just be in a position to negotiate, but would have to, knowing that they are paying part of their medical expenses themselves. They would have to be more discerning not just in their choice of doctors, but also show more interest in their treatment plans with part of the costs of consultation, prescriptions, lab, hospitalizations, and other such bills coming directly from their pockets. Under these circumstances, is it not only fair, and indeed, absolutely necessary, to provide healthcare consumers with the necessary information to make such choices? With respect to seniors, who constitute a significant percentage of healthcare consumers, and their numbers likely to increase in future as baby-boomers turn seniors, and beyond, is it not even more necessary considering that they have much less money to expend on healthcare? In the U.S, for example, do they not need to have as much information as possible for example on the Medicare Prescription Part D prescription drug benefit that became effective January 1, 2006, for example regarding the Centers for Medicare and Medicaid Services (CMS) approved drug plans, hence to decide which one to enroll with? Should seniors not know the latest regarding Medicaid coverage of prescription drugs for Medicare beneficiaries, the so-called dual-eligibles, and if they have not chosen a plan, to which randomly assigned automatically, particularly with enrollment period ending in Mid-May 2006? Should they not know the drugs plans cover, and billing arrangements, and other such relevant information? Does the fact that our seniors currently and even more so in future are computer savvy, in the main, not offer us immense opportunities to create programs targeted at seniors, using a variety of healthcare ICT that would provide them with the necessary information to make those choices, and should we not already be thinking about such programs? Would there be competition with the players, this time, the healthcare providers, not knowing what their competitors are charging for similar services? How could we expect prices to fall and overall healthcare costs to drop without such competition, and other market forces operational? How would seniors, and indeed others who must spend a portion of their own resources on deductibles and co-payments know which healthcare provider is more cost-effective? As we have noted in our discussion, healthcare faces serious challenges in most countries, not least what to do about soaring costs, and declining quality. In fact, healthcare is going to be more important as time goes on, and some would argue, it is heading for center-stage in our world. What is also doing the same is the interplay of competitive forces in healthcare delivery, regardless of the funding of the health system. So long as someone has to pay for health services, we are all stakeholders in the business, and it does not matter who is paying, and where the funds are coming from. Even if employers for example, manage to cut down health benefits, and/or automate all their operations, who would buy their products? Should we expect ill people prostrate in bed to go shopping? Would families struggling to save up enough to purchase health coverage have enough to spare for electronics, and cars? What would happen to the overall economy if people saved up rather than spend their money? Perhaps we should take a cue from Japan, and how long it took its peoples to start to spend money again, and what could have happened to the country's economy if they did not recently? So, health plays crucial roles on both the supply and demand sides, and this has nothing to do with its funding? Even in a publicly funded system, the country would either have to trim the health services it offers its peoples or tax them more to fund an increasingly pricey health system. Before long, it would find itself in a catch 22 situation, with excessive trimming of services resulting in an unhealthier populace, and increasing taxes likely to create discontent in the end among the peoples, particularly in an aging population where fewer and fewer would have to bear the tax burden. This is why even such systems need to acknowledge the need to act now to avoid this situation. We all need to start with the dual objectives of delivering qualitative healthcare, simultaneously reducing healthcare costs. Of course, we could decide to ignore the latter, but at what costs, and should we not use the resources that we have and could continue to improve upon to prevent healthcare costs escalating to the point that we now see the need for action to stop it increasing further? Incidentally, healthcare ICT, which is the third prong of the center-stage tripartite, is all around us, offering opportunities to develop innovative programs to improve the processes involved in healthcare delivery. This is another important concept that we need to appreciate, that is that healthcare delivery is a complex arrangement of processes from clinical, administrative, supplies, management, and finance, among others, the overall efficiency of which would result in the achievement of our dual objectives. These processes involve acquisition, storage, transmission, sharing, and others, including decision support, and actionable policy formulation. The more efficient these various processes and activities are, the likelier would be our chances of achieving our goals. Which is more efficient for example, between sending a document that would lead to an urgent, perhaps, even mission-critical, actionable decision via snail or electronically? We need to start to see the immense opportunities healthcare ICT offers us in meeting the challenges that healthcare delivery pose now and would pose in the years ahead, for example, when baby-boomers turn seniors in five years. Only then would we be able to see which processes what technology would buoy its efficiency, and not therefore be mismatching, implementing healthcare ICT. Again, we need to remember that we set out to achieve two broad objectives. This means that we must consider other aspects of the tripartite, healthcare delivery, and competitive forces. In fact, the three parts of the centerpiece of our lives work together in unison, changes to one likely to influence one or more of the others, the overall effect the determinant of the success or otherwise of our quest to achieve the dual objectives. Each of these prongs has its own subsystem, again all impinging on one another to create the overall effect of the particular prong. Let us consider healthcare delivery for example. The state of medical knowledge, the prevalence and distribution patterns of diseases, health indicators of various kinds, culture, service utilization, and its associated factors such as insurance coverage levels, and the expectations of the end users, inextricably linked with the quality of service provision, for examples determine singly or in combination what healthcare delivery looks like in any country. They do not do so exclusively, however, because the two other prongs mentioned earlier and their subsystems impinge on healthcare delivery too. It is easier to tackle some of these issues than others, depending of course on which point of view one holds. It might be easier for some for example to urge the need to define parameters in working out the required policies for preventing healthcare costs soaring, with the taxpayer not having to be responsible for others' actions when they should not? In other words, to advocate the need for the health consumer to be responsible for part of his/her treatment costs in the U.S, for example, than in Canada, which runs privately, and publicly, funded health systems, respectively.

To be sure, the health consumer in even publicly funded health systems such as in

Canada, pays for health services that Medicare does not cover, their numbers and types varying from one province to another. The point is that even when the health consumer pays part of his/her healthcare costs, the efforts would likely not achieve the desired objectives of making health consumers more discerning in their choices not only of doctors, but also of lifestyles within a health system of persistent information asymmetry for instance. With regard, publicly funded systems, could anyone argue that considering that reports have it that Canadians are willing to pay more to keep the Medicare status quo, that they would not eventually have to be just as discerning, which in fact they already are. Would they not be demanding higher quality health services for their money, just as their counterparts in the U.S? Would this not put the onus on their providers, for examples, GPs, to deliver such services, or lose their clientele? With the increasing push toward ambulatory/community/domiciliary services, would even regional health hospitals not increasingly need to justify their very existence if they could not provide the expected services? Are competitive forces not already at play even in such publicly funded health systems, given this scenario? Would these competitive forces not ultimately play out among GPs, family doctors, and even among specialists in the hospitals that survive? Why would patients not seek out their elective surgeries in hospital X in town Y if the surgeon in hospital J, in town K, where they live is not as competent as the former, based on information gleaned from doctors' profile made public, to facilitate more discernible decision-making on choice of doctors by the consumer? Would this not affect the fortunes of the latter surgeon, and his/her hospital's, and would both not have to do something to improve their standing, and is this not competition? The question then is what role healthcare ICT would play in how these competitive forces play out, and what should we do to exploit the opportunities that these technologies offer in fostering such competition? Consider also the issue of service utilization. Many would not contend the likelihood of someone overusing health services if he or she would not have to pay for them. Yet, this sort of abuse of the health system is responsible for a significant portion of the soaring healthcare costs again regardless of the health system's funding structure. Could healthcare ICT also help in tackling this problem? Do we need to educate people on these issues, do these issues highlight the need for cost sharing in healthcare delivery, and to what extent should this be? We are going to have to start thinking outside the box, literally, in our approach to health education and disease prevention, both in terms of form and content in order to make significant strides in reducing healthcare costs and keeping people healthy. It is going to require a delicate balancing act to promote healthy exercising including sporting activities, for example, while simultaneously discouraging deliberate involvement in activities that are inimical to health, if not even survival, for example, going skiing when there are clear avalanche warnings. Some would contend that in a publicly funded health system such as in Canada, this could only mean provinces and territories further limiting coverage, but this does not have to be the case. Firstly, everyone is and should continue to be free to seek treatment in an ER department, as is the case even in a privately funded health system such as in the U.S. The question is what happens after this initial emergency treatment? Should the defined parameters mentioned above now come into force? Some would answer in the affirmative and ask that with extensive prior consultations with the public, healthcare providers, other healthcare stakeholders, and thorough economic analyses of diseases, among other considerations, if we could not arrive at feasible arrangements regarding coverage, and its extent in costs and duration. There is no doubt about this idea already implemented perhaps based on different assumptions in Canada, and elsewhere, as Medicare does not cover every health problem as noted above, but there is also no doubt about the challenges such moves would pose to entrenched values in the Canadian society, which would make implementing such an arrangements arduous, even if doable. Indeed, an article in the May 09, 2006, Volume 42, Issue 17, of the Medical Post has suggested may be it was time we revisited "the tax-based model". The article noted in particular that Dr. Dennis Furlong, in his 2004 book, Medicare Myths: 50 Myths We've Endured about the Canadian Health Care System, presented the concept of a prorated patient contribution (PPC) model, which essentially advocated for Canadians, except the most financially-challenged, to pay unstipulated and varying graduated amounts on their healthcare, based on taxable income. According to the doctor, "Patients should actively participate in the costs of their individual care." Many indeed, would agree with the doctor that the health system is over-used, and that is unsustainable, considering its cost implications. The questions remain though, if instituting a parallel private health system is the answer, or it is requesting Canadians to pay for some of their healthcare costs, which with regard the latter the Romanow Report noted that Canadians are willing to pay a little more to help defend the public system. Dr Furlong suggested all but the poorest Canadians would put in new, prorated shares of their incomes to government revenues devoted to health care, a similar measure in the 2002 Kirby report that some considered a user fee, and essentially seemingly avoided by most policy analysts. Some would however, argue that we could not avoid this matter for too long considering the ever-increasing costs of healthcare delivery in the country, an increase that would likely be even more as more Canadians become seniors. Given these facts, and the tripartite relationships between healthcare delivery, competition, and healthcare ICT mentioned earlier, could we make healthcare more affordable and qualitative, while containing costs? Could fostering competition, even in a publicly funded health system, and promoting ICT diffusion, and encouraging all healthcare stakeholders to embrace and implement these technologies help us achieve these goals? The House of Commons passed the Canada Health Act in 1984, unanimously and by all accounts, many Canadians want the health system to remain publicly funded, and indeed, Alberta recently had to jettison its "Third Way" healthcare delivery model, which had significant private care input. However, Quebec and British Columbia are pressing ahead with their versions of a parallel private health system. Considering the Quebec Supreme Court decision mentioned earlier, some argue that it is a matter of time before the other provinces would also have to allow its residents the option of seeking private healthcare, but this for now is conjectural. So then, how could competition and healthcare ICT help us achieve our goals in a publicly funded system such as in Canada? Let us start with what we do with information, the common denominator in healthcare industry transactions. To underscore the importance of rectifying the information asymmetry mentioned earlier, the European Commission (EU) on May 10, 2006 launched a Europe-wide Internet portal that aims to provide citizens and professionals with information on health-related issues. The website, located at http://health.europa.eu has 47 topics on a variety of issues including on alcohol problems, babies' health, bio-terrorism, and vaccinations, has links to information on health policies of member states and to the websites of European non-governmental agencies and those of international organizations, and provides indicators and statistics on health across the continent. The EU also expects the website, which provides information in the EU's 20 current official languages, to serve as a veritable research portal for policy makers, healthcare professionals, and scientists, and indeed, anyone seeking information on healthcare delivery in the EU. There are in fact fundamental reasons why we need information, and it does not matter in what type of society we are. There is no doubt about the role language has played in our lives as humans. Indeed, one dare says that we might not still be on this planet, even barring any natural catastrophe, had we not developed language. Put differently, language has been the key to our advancement to where we are today as humans, and has made us outsmart every other living creature on this planet, at least known to us. In fact, one could say that it was inevitable that we did since we have language. Language has proven to be the most potent communication medium, far superior to pheromones, or other communication mechanisms between living things, and communication is the operational word here. Language only has value in communication, which could be verbal or non-verbal. Just as language gave us a competitive edge over other living things, even those far larger, and more physically stronger than we are, it is what confers competitive advantage among us humans. The crucial factor is the efficiency of its usage, after all, animals also communicate in some form or another, but our mode of communication seems to be the most efficient, hence our superiority over these other beings. The point here is that language is the machinery of communication, information, its raw material, and action, its product. Without information therefore, language is useless, and there would be no action, or decision. Without action, there is no new information and nothing for language to express or process, hence no further decision, or action, and eventually, the machinery undergoes disuse atrophy, and the language becomes moribund, and dies. With the death of the language is the entire organism, or possibly even civilization. The use of language therefore not only confers competitive advantage but it is imperative for survival. Thus, survival is the underlying principle of language. In other words, language exists for us to survive, and indeed, for any living being to survive, language, as competition earlier, conceptualized, generically, as a means of information expression and communication. We would not need language were we able to survive sitting quietly in one location, living a stress-free existence, everyt hing we need within reach, and we have no need to protect ourselves from anyone, or anything, even the elements. Even then, ants would probably devour us in the real state of affairs in our world, if some more enterprising and agile predator did not get to us first. Language has made it possible for us to communicate with our fellow beings and take collective actions even in our prehistoric days regarding imminent danger, or where food, shelter, and water were, and in our travels, and dispersal all over the globe. We have succeeded as a species because we could use information, and compete against other living beings and one another, as individuals, and as whole societies. Information communication and sharing have led to increased efficiency of the processes inherent in our activities crucial to our survival, hence to individual and societal progress. This means that the more efficient our communication is, the more efficient these processes are, and the more progress we would make. Many of the societal institutions, religious, legal, political, financial, and medical, for examples, that we have today were great works in communication nurtured by language. These works constitute the basis of modern society, and continue to influence our moral, ethical, political, and economic thoughts, and the direction humanity heads. Therefore, it makes intuitive sense for us to continue to create, communicate, and use information, in the most efficient and effective ways to forge ahead. This is where, in the medical realm, the use of healthcare ICT becomes crucial, as these technologies would make our information communication and sharing more efficient, hence facilitate more rational and proficient decision making. It is clear from our discussion so far that information communication and competition are flipsides of the same coin, ICT, the bridge linking them. Thus, without information, there is no competition, and without competition, information becomes redundant, even useless. If we applied this analysis to healthcare delivery, what would be the purpose of the immense information store in health if we could not communicate and share it among healthcare providers, and other healthcare stakeholders? What is the purpose of sharing the information, if it were not to give us some advantage, for example, in preventing disease, or treating a patient, or choosing the best doctor? Would choosing or method over another in all these three instances not amount to competition, since there is a preference? Is the prospect of such preference not likely to stimulate interest in developing ways to make better choices? Would the scientists working on vaccines in different companies, for example, not work harder to ensure choosing theirs? Would this not make for more qualitative prevention tools? Armed with the best prevention, would we not more likely survive the disease posing a threat to us, for example, avian flu, and what would be the effect of the lack of such success on our overall health, that of our industries, and businesses, and on the economies of countries, even the global economy? Could we not have prevented this catastrophe simply using information more efficiently deploying appropriate healthcare ICT? Do these competitive processes have anything to do with the funding structure of the health system? Should we not in fact encourage such competitive processes in both publicly and privately funded health systems, contextually? Besides the health benefits of the vaccine production example mentioned earlier, is not that we would not only be able to purchase the best vaccines available but the prices of vaccines would fall, due to the operations of market forces, and would such measures not help us contain overall healthcare costs, with more firms engaged in producing vaccines? What we are driving at is that competition is an integral aspect of our lives, and indeed, necessary for our survival, and that healthcare ICT could enhance it, and both applied to healthcare delivery, could make it possible, and easier, to achieve our dual objectives of delivering qualitative healthcare, cost-effectively, irrespective of the funding model of the healthcare system. The nature and extent of competition would be situation-specific, no doubt, in particular, in details, and modus operandi, but it is competition, all the same and it is with the appropriate healthcare ICT implemented, enhanced as is healthcare delivery improved. Should every country, therefore, not be seeking the best ways to exploit the opportunities that healthcare ICT offers in improving its health services? Is this not the more urgent were we to sustain the levels of quality of current healthcare delivery, let alone, improve it, particularly considering the likely further increases in healthcare costs as baby-boomers turn seniors in the next five years, and the population ages still further in the developed, and even the developing countries? To be sure, the changing disease patterns, health indicators, progress in medical knowledge, and in technological development, and of a variety of socio-economic, cultural, and ethico-moral factors, mentioned above as subsystems of healthcare delivery, are going to require a constant reappraisal of healthcare coverage, even in publicly funded health systems. This is more so that competitive forces and healthcare ICT are going to be exerting their push and pull in a milieu of finite resources. To under the need for such reappraisal and that of information in the process, consider a recent study by Finnish researchers published in the May 13, 2006 issue of the British Medical Journal. The researchers noted that we might be heading in the wrong direction seeking inherited genes that increase people's risks for cancer, genes that the researchers said that might not exist. The researchers noted that that if such genes existed, they would not likely have much effect on the incidence of cancer, on which in fact they noted studies show environmental, dietary or lifestyle changes have a much larger effect than do genes. The researchers even contend that the strong link between specific genes and increased cancer risks might be flawed. They also observed that the changes these studies found in the incidence of cancer within one generation or two generations simply occurred to quickly for their cause to be the intrusion of new genes. Such studies include twin studies that showed that genetic vulnerability played a small-to-moderate role in the incidence of cancer. The researchers admitted that certain genes might increase cancer risk in specific instances, such as the BRCA1 and BRCA2 genes and breast cancer risk, but not cancer in general. How would we be able to evaluate our understanding of cancers, and indeed, other diseases, hence be able to manage them better without this sort of information, and would we have the information without promoting research activities, which are themselves subject to competitive forces in the academia? Does this study not also point to the need for more energetic primary prevention efforts to control the environmental factors that seem to be crucial to our developing many diseases, efforts that healthcare ICT could play a major role in helping ensure their success? Is it not deducible from this study that we need public policies to help develop appropriate initiatives to actualize these primary prevention programs? Would we not be able to achieve our dual goals starting these programs now that could reduce morbidities and mortalities in seniors, current, and in those baby-boomers that would soon become seniors, and indeed, in everyone else? Should the public also not have this information, particularly those with a family history of cancer? A recent U.S study published in the May 2006 issue of *Carcinogenesis* for example reported that exercise might help reduce the risk of skin cancer, which buttresses the need for us to intensify preventive measures, many simple, and inexpensive, and even more so, and more effective backed by healthcare ICT, in battling cancer and other diseases for that matter. The researchers at Rutgers University exposed female mice to a form of ultraviolet light, and noticed that the mice took longer to develop skin tumors if they had access to a running wheel. They also found that exercise seemed to accelerate the rate at which cancer cells die, although cautioned that their findings were no reason for indiscriminate and unprotected outings in the sun. The researchers exposed the mice to ultraviolet B (UVB) thrice a week for 16 weeks during the study's first part termed, the high risk model, ten for the next 14 weeks, without further UVB treatment, gave half the mice access to running wheels in their cages, but not the other half. They exposed the mice to UVB light twice a week for 33 weeks, and, from the start, only 50% had access to a running wheel, in the second part of the study. The results: all the mice in the high-risk model developed skin tumors, within 7, and 3.5 weeks, for the mice that exercised, and those that did not, respectively, the tumors in the former, also less numerous and smaller. The decrease in non-malignant tumor size per mouse was by 54% and malignant tumor size per mouse, by 73%. The results of the study's second part were similar, the exercising mice slower to develop tumors, and had fewer and smaller tumors, non-malignant tumor size per mouse decreased by 75%, malignant tumor size per mouse by 69%. On analyzing the samples, the researchers discovered that exercise seemed to enhance programmed cell death (apoptosis), which removes sun-damaged cells in both skin and tumors, negating the tumor development UVB causes. The researchers also found that mice with less fat developed fewer tumors, a key point considering the increasing, if not epidemic prevalence of obesity worldwide, particularly in the developed countries. Should we not let people have this sort of information? Would it not help increase awareness of the possible risk for skin cancer of obesity, too, and the role of exercise, which indeed other studies have shown that along with a healthy diet, could help reduce the risk of several cancer types? Should we not strongly emphasize in giving the public the information that it is no excuse for going exercising in the hot sun without proper protection considering that the sun's UV rays are a major cause of skin cancer, and that we should, particularly the fair complexioned, avoid the rays particularly when the sun is most intense? Does these studies not speak to the need for targeted, contextualized health information delivered to those that need it, rather than expecting them to search for it, which many might not do, considering our busy and tension-soaked, contemporary existence? Besides the information on many of the Internet health sites for example, being dated and inaccurate, some slant toward the information provider's marketing needs. Besides, health consumers are increasingly wary of search engines, as some lead users to websites that change their browser setting and redirect them to ad sites or expose them to spam, spyware and other perilous downloads, simply typing in an innocuous keyword.

As noted earlier, not only do genes have strong links with increased risk of certain

cancers, they also do with other diseases, as the following recent findings on coronary heart disease show. Researchers at the National Institute of Environmental Health Sciences found that a common genetic variation increase some people's susceptibility to coronary heart disease (CHD). The report noted that Caucasians that have this gene variation are about 1.5 times likelier to have a CHD event, for example, a heart attack, than those that do not, and roughly, 15% of them have this specific gene variation, or polymorphisms. According to Craig Lee, Pharm.D, a researcher at NIEHS and lead author on the study, published in the Volume 15, No. 10 issue of "Human Molecular Genetics", "We found that Caucasians who carry this

polymorphism, named K55R, were at significantly higher risk of coronary heart disease, independent of other risk factors, like cigarette smoking, diabetes, and hypertension. We did not observe the same association in African Americans who had the K55R polymorphism." The research indicates that Caucasians with this polymorphism break down quite rapidly, beneficial fatty acids termed

epoxyeicosatrienoic acids, or EETs, known to play a protective role in the cardiovascular system, for examples, lowering blood pressure, preventing blood clotting, and combating inflammation. The K55R polymorphism is an inherited variation of "EPHX2", which latter generates an enzyme that eliminates beneficial EET fatty acids from the body during metabolism, this normal process, thus, accelerated in persons with the K55R polymorphism, with more of the protective

EETs therefore lost. Not only does this study underscore this gene's significance in heart diseases and in identifying persons at high risk, but also the possible value of this metabolic pathway in targeting preventive strategies for preventing these diseases. With coronary heart disease being a major public health problem, about 1.2 million Americans estimated to experience a CHD event in 2006 alone, there is no doubt about the significance of such studies as these and the need to let those who need to know their findings do so. That researches such as these update our medical knowledge is an important aspect of our efforts to improve the quality of healthcare delivery, and indeed, to promote competition in helping us do so, the third prong of the tripartite mentioned above. The deployment of the appropriate technologies to ensure the dissemination of the new knowledge to those that need it as described above is also crucial in the interplay of factors that result in our achievement of the dual objectives also mentioned earlier. Consider another recent research study published in "Science" on May 05, 2006, on the neurobiology of dread. This new research, perhaps the first brain imaging study of dread, which the National Institute on Drug Abuse (NIDA), National Institutes of Health supported, indicated that it is possible to tell individuals that experience significant dread regarding adverse events biologically from those that tolerate them better. The ramifications of this study include enabling better understanding of how the brains of non-addicted individuals decide on actions to take in unpleasant circumstances and outcomes, which open the door, literally to understanding how the brains of individuals that use/abuse illicit substances, for examples, and that have other "addictive" behaviors or drive disorders, make such choices. As NIH Director, Dr. Elias Zerhouni noted, "Brain imaging technology offers unique insight into the biological mechanisms involved in decision-making, which is invaluable in developing tailored treatment strategies for addiction and drug abuse." Would this not help in reducing the prevalence of this problem in society, and by extension, the burden of the disease on the individuals concerned, and their families, not to mention the reduction in healthcare costs that would likely follow? Understanding for example, that drug abusers place more value on short-rather than long-term outcomes, as previous research evidence has shown would assist in designing the appropriate psychological therapies for these individuals, whose chances of success such understanding would enhance. The researchers in this study used functional magnetic resonance imaging (fMRI) to create images of brain activity in 32 nondrug-abusing participants expecting brief pedal electrical shocks. They charted the regions that had increased blood flow over time, hence were able to figure the link between certain mental activities and specific brain areas. The researchers noted that activity patterns linked with the dread of waiting involved brain areas that govern our perception of pain. Specifically, the responses occurred in brain areas attention, more than those fear seemingly govern. The researchers also determined each participant's maximal pain threshold, each then given a series of choices from 36 possibilities, ranging from choosing to receive a shock 30% of their threshold in 27 seconds or one, 60% in 9 seconds. According to Dr. Gregory Berns of Emory University School of Medicine, one of the researchers, "We noted that normal, healthy subjects could be divided into two groups --extreme dreaders, who could not tolerate a delay and preferred an immediate (and stronger) painful stimulus; and mild dreaders, who could tolerate a delay for a milder shock." He added, "We saw that the extreme dreaders could be distinguished from the mild dreaders by virtue of the information captured on the brain scans. The findings suggest that dread derives, in part, from the attention devoted to the expected physical response and is not simply a fear or anxiety reaction." Commenting on the findings, another researcher Dr. Volkow noted, "Continuing to use drugs despite the expectation of the practice's negative effects is a hallmark of addiction" "The results of this study form the foundation for future research to determine whether drug abusers exhibit disruption in the brain systems that process the anticipation of unpleasant consequences". What could better understanding dread offer us in the palliative care of seniors for example, besides its benefits in the management of addictive behaviors, for example, alcohol dependence, which is relatively common among the elderly? The above examples illustrate the complex interactions between information generation and communication, the technologies that facilitate these processes, and the competitive forces that underpin them, in improving healthcare delivery, and in reducing healthcare costs. It is clear, based on our discussion so far that the achievement of these dual objectives is feasible, but we need to have the proper conceptualizations of the issues involved in so doing, in particular the significance of competition, as a rallying focus. It is important for us to recognize the role competition plays in not only stimulating technological creativity and innovation, but in also fostering research efforts that culminate in new medical knowledge, and a better understanding of diseases and healthcare delivery processes. We should also recognize the role that healthcare ICT plays in promoting competition, thereby making healthcare delivery more accessible, and affordable, and perhaps most importantly, more qualitative. An understanding of the dynamics between these tripartite factors is the fundamental premise from which detailed initiatives in achieving the dual objectives would spring, and this is irrespective of but contextual to the funding structure of the health system in question. To illustrate the epigenetic nature of forces working in concert to help us achieve these dual objectives, consider the recent agreement between British Prime Minister Tony Blair, and the country's Chancellor of the Exchequer, Gordon Brown on pensions policies, under which, the restoration of the link between the state pension and earnings will occur, probably in 2012. This would be two years after the date recommended by Lord Turner's commission on pensions. The deal reached on May 11, 2006, also involved increasing the state pension age raised to 68 years, by 2050, the shift to a more generous state pension, and avoidance of large tax increases, and described as "affordable" by government, the shadow chancellor George Osborne, embraced,

despite misgivings by many in the Opposition. In 2005, Lord Turner published his report, in which he recommended raising the state pension age from 65 to 68 by 2050 to help handle the mounting costs linked with an increasingly aging population, healthcare delivery a significant cost driver. Lord Turner also called for the state pension to be more munificent, with increases from 2010 linked to average wages and not price inflation, the former, pensions advocates have long sought. In Lord Turner's view, delaying retirement age and utilizing the funds saved with women's pension age synchronized with men's between 2010 and 2020, would pay for restoring the link with average earnings, which Margaret Thatcher's government broke in 1980. Reacting to the deal mentioned above, pensions experts believe that the state pension will still be there but would be of less significance in terms of people's overall income in retirement. If this were so, what would its ramifications be for health services delivery to seniors in the U.K? Would government have more money to provide health services in a health system that is taxation-based, and what would the likelihood of more tax revenues portend for the disposable income of the seniors and would having to work three years longer have beneficial or adverse health consequences? On the other hand, would this deal run aground with the funds to execute it lacking, or would government have to increase taxes? These are questions whose answers are critical to the success or otherwise of the agreement mentioned above, and to the future of healthcare delivery, to seniors, and indeed, to everyone else in the U.K. With the population of other developed countries also aging, should part of planning for the likely increases in healthcare costs that would occur in future not be revisiting the pension issue? With this issue, we see again, the competition subsystem at work in determining the future of healthcare delivery, seniors having to work, hence remain in the competitive free-market, for an extra three years, this competitiveness having a direct effect on possible resource availability, most likely positively considering the revenue generation from taxes from those additional years. This is even more so considering that the seniors would still have been able to receive free healthcare in the NHS even if otherwise retired in those three years anyway. Furthermore, with intensive healthcare ICT backed health education and disease prevention programs, the inevitable more exposure to physical activity, and continuing availability of, if not more disposable income to afford the things that spice up their lives, hence enhancing its quality, we might be able to reduce or delay the onset of certain ailments in these seniors. The extra working years might thus offer an opportunity to in fact, spend less on the seniors' health down the road. Again, we see the possible interactions between the tripartite systems mentioned earlier in helping us achieve the dual objectives also mentioned earlier. The theme of our discussion thus far has been the vital role that competition and healthcare ICT play in healthcare delivery, regardless of the health system and that an appreciation of these factors' interplay with healthcare delivery offers, us a veritable channel for actualizing our goals of delivering qualitative healthcare to the populace cost-effectively. This appreciation involves decomposing the tripartite systems into subsystems, understanding how the subsystems interact with one another and with the other subsystems to create the overall systems interplay that result eventually in the achievement of our set goals. As we have repeatedly emphasized thus far, one of the key aspects of our efforts toward achieving these goals is rectifying the information asymmetry that has been the bane of the health industry for so long. With the paradigm shift in the industry toward consumer-oriented healthcare delivery model, the resolve to make information available to the healthcare consumer becomes in fact, imperative. The healthcare consumer is also the focal point in other health systems for example in the U.K and Canada, even if they do not call their healthcare delivery models the same name, or indeed, fund their systems similarly as in the U.S.. Wherever the patient takes center stage in the healthcare delivery scheme, the need for the consumer to have relevant, accurate and current health information is not only desirable, as it is in fact even otherwise, but just as imperative. The healthcare consumer should not only be able to receive information on wellness and a variety of diseases that interest him/her, but also information that would enable the comparisons of costs and quality, both elements of competition, acting differently, and in tandem with healthcare ICT for example, in determining choice. Healthcare ICT for example, might be responsible for the quality of service provision that attracts consumers to a particular doctor and not another, or it might just be the human touch or some personality characteristics of the doctor that fosters the doctor-patient relationship, despite the doctor's prices being higher than those of his/her peers. This example shows the interplay of the elements of the subsystems mentioned above, and the need to understand these interplays as best as we could in order to be able to formulate policies more rationally, and deploy initiatives more effectively. We need to continue to make pricing information public for example to be more useful. Some contend for example prices hospitals, doctors and private data companies often predicate on average, not specific to any hospital, or other measures such as what insurers paid for the services, prices that are sometimes currently irrelevant. This is considering for example that health plans negotiate discounts off the list prices, and that the information for those with insurance coverage might not apply to their specific policies, although the uninsured might be able to glean something from the information that would help him/her. For the realization of the full benefits on the U.S. health system of the increasing interest of employers in offering workers higher deductible coverage, for example, the consumer needs information to make the right choices. The present U.S. administration under President Bush has endorsed such high-deductible coverage, which consumers could use with health savings accounts, enabling them to save money tax-free for their future healthcare costs, measures with the potential to promote price information and, reduce healthcare costs as consumers take better care in using their funds on healthcare. However, they need price and quality information to make these choices, and healthcare ICT could assist in delivering this information to the healthcare consumer, cost-effectively. With prices down, health coverage would be more affordable for more Americans or would they? Some contend that high-deductible plans would only interest the healthy and those with the funds to purchase them, and would do little to reduce health spending even with information readily available. Others argue that this might be in the short-term but that overall, these plans would deliver the expected results. With more efforts at encouraging not just the health industry, but insurers and other key players in healthcare delivery to make pricing and quality data and information available publicly, there is no doubt that the initial skews in the free-market operations some worry about would dissipate as the numbers of buyer and sellers increase significantly. Indeed, this seems to have started happening, with enrollment in high-deductible plans that qualify for health savings accounts (HSA) tripling to three million in 10 months, according to a study released on January 26, 2006, by America's Health Insurance Plans. The study, based on responses from AHIP member firms, including nearly every one of them that offers HSA-eligible plans, showed that the market for HSAs is enlarging as companies make them available in more markets and to a broader range of large and small groups, and to individual healthcare consumers. In short, people are getting used to HSAs more than ever before, increasing the prospects of the plans achieving their expected goals, although more still need to sign up, as currently enrollees still amounts to only a small percentage of Americans who have private insurance, 198 million of them, privately insured. Some would even argue that perhaps an even greater expansion of the plans is apt in order to encourage further more of those with comprehensive health insurance to make more cost-effective health care decisions, the central vision of the consumer-driven health system. The recent foray of financial systems into the health industry also exemplifies the operations of the competition subsystems, and how they affect healthcare delivery, a phenomenon more of which we are likely to see in the years ahead. Banks, money managers, and credit unions, for examples, are increasingly perched to play central roles in healthcare delivery via the health savings accounts (HSA) unable to resist the lure of the significant profits they could make offering healthcare consumers mutual funds, with the growth of their account balances. These financial institutions charge roughly $50, some slightly more, to open an HSA, plus another about $40 annual service fees, an increasing number of such institutions now in the HSA business, which accounts they make money from even without investment management fees, simply from payment processing when a consumer uses his/her HSA debit card at a doctor's office. Some experts estimate that just another four years, about 10% of all those insured Americans would have an HSA, the banks making billion of dollars in payment processing alone during the same period. Would the healthcare consumer also make profits from the mutual funds, for example, that would enlarge their HSA balances, hence make healthcare even more affordable, or would the financial institutions eat the profits and even their HSAs up in processing fees? What effect would the latter have on the ability of the healthcare consumer to afford coverage? Would the healthcare consumer be able to transfer accounts based on information obtained on the quality of services the financial institutions provide, including on the performance of their funds portfolios? There are thus elements in the competition subsystem some directly related to the health system, others not, that could play crucial roles in the direction and quality of healthcare delivery, which elements we need to analyze thoroughly in order to fully understand the behavior and ramifications of the competitive forces both at play. We need to know these factors at play now, and those that would likely be at play in the years ahead in determining healthcare delivery quality, and costs, which would facilitate policy formulation, and resource planning and allocation to confront the tasks of healthcare provision ahead, for examples regarding our seniors, successfully.

The healthcare ICT subsystems are also key players in healthcare delivery, and we could decompose them into smaller interactive components and factors. As the major facilitators of the competitive processes in healthcare delivery, the more healthcare stakeholders also implement and use them, the better functioning the competitive processes are, and the higher our chances of achieving the dual objectives of delivering qualitative health cost-effectively mentioned earlier. Patient safety is one key healthcare quality parameter. Yet, hospitals and healthcare providers in general, have tended to be somewhat reluctant to disclose such information as infection rates, medical errors, and other relevant patient safety information. Consumers also need such information to make the correct choices about healthcare providers. Efforts ought to continue in encouraging providers to disclose such information, again, to ensure the smooth running of the competitive processes necessary to improve the quality of healthcare delivery, including the implementation of the appropriate technologies to help improve patient safety. Healthcare ICT for example, is helping reduce medical error rates, and there is recent evidence for this assertion from two new studies from the Johns Hopkins Children's Center that showed that computerizing ordering of chemotherapy and other forms of intravenous drug infusions for children significantly reduces the risk of medical errors. Christoph Lehmann, M.D., director of clinical information technology at the Children's Center, and his team developed the online infusion calculator and a computerized drug ordering system already in use for three years, but whose effect on medical errors they only just measured. With children thrice at risk for medication errors than adults, due essentially to the often complicated ordering and dosing regimes they need, including the need to calculate dosing based on age, height and weight, miscalculations and rounding errors are rife and could be potentially fatal. This is even more so as children's still-developing systems have less tolerance for drug over dosages and the like. According to Lehman, lead author of the Web-based calculator study, published in the May 2006 issue of *Pediatric Critical Care Medicine,* "Our findings reveal that using a Web-based calculator makes it less likely to order and give a child the wrong dose or commit other errors, such as omitting patient information, weight parameters, or infusion rates". He added, "Our calculator stops ordering errors before they can even reach the pharmacy, let alone the patient. "The calculator computes all doses. It also advises and alerts doctors on drug interactions, offering "default" doses, and drug dilutions automatically to assist them in averting over-and under-dosing. The researchers compared handwritten and calculator-generated orders prior to and after using the online calculator, 27% of the former wrong, with an error rate of 45 errors per every 100 such orders, 94% of the latter, correct, the error rate, just 6 per 100. Most handwritten errors were wrong dosage and wrong concentration, both high-risk errors, not one of which the calculator-generated orders had. In order to evaluate the effect of the computerized physician order entry (CPOE) system on pediatric chemotherapy orders, the researchers compared 1,259 handwritten to 1,116 electronic orders. The results showed that CPOE-based orders had fewer cumulative dose omissions, and dose miscalculations, were less likely to have incomplete nurse safety checklists, and averted 17 to 18 such errors per every 100-drug orders. The drug order system uses calculators that adjust dosage to the patient's age and weight, automatically, thus making complicated calculations unnecessary, and the risk of calculation errors much less, doctors indeed, essentially compelled to select options from a dropdown menu hence preventing handwriting orders. The authors cautioned that despite their successes, human input in ensuring safety is also important, and recommend adopting automated systems for intravenous drug infusions, and drug orders, particularly in pediatric oncology units, pediatric ICU, and ERs, all known high-risk areas, and indeed recommended the adoption of these technologies in all areas of medicine. There is no doubt about the need for such healthcare ICT diffusion, which as we discussed earlier, would foster competitiveness, improve healthcare delivery, and eventually help reduce healthcare costs. Still on patient safety, a recent Agency for Healthcare Research and Quality and Research (AHRQ) study, "Reducing Warfarin Medication Interaction: An Interrupted Time Series Evaluation," published in the May 8, 2006 issue of *Archives of Internal Medicine*

found that computer alerts could help reduce the rate doctors prescribe drugs capable of interacting with blood thinners. The researchers ordered 15% less prescriptions for such drugs as Warfarin, using a computerized system that signals a safety alert whenever doctors key in the name of the interacting drug. If a doctor in one of 15 primary care clinics used a computerized system to prescribe one of five potentially interacting drugs to a patient taking warfarin, namely acetaminophen, non-steroidal ant-inflammatory drugs, fluconazole, metronidazole, or sulfamethoxasole, an alert showed up on the screen signaling the potential hazard, and suggested substitute drugs. When the study commenced in December 2002, doctors prescribed 3,294 interacting drugs per 10,000 patients receiving warfarin, but only 2,804, at its end in March 2003. Despite increasing evidence of the value of healthcare ICT, these technologies are yet to be widely accepted even in many developed countries, including Canada and the U.S. The findings of a recent study give us an insight into improving acceptance of computerized prescribing alerts in ambulatory care[11]. The study noted that poor specificity and alert overload are some of the reasons for overriding computerized drug prescribing alerts. The researchers set out to improve clinician acceptance of drug alerts by designing a selective set of drug alerts for the ambulatory care setting. They minimized workflow disruptions by allowing only critical to high-severity alerts to interrupt clinician workflow. The researchers presented the alerts to clinicians using computerized prescribing within an electronic medical record (EMR) in 31 Boston-area practices, generating 18,115 drug alerts during the study's six-month period, 12,933 (71%), noninterruptive, 5,182 (29%), interruptive, 67% of the latter, accepted. Reasons for overrides for each drug alert category were not uniform, and offered valuable information for improving alerts. The authors concluded that their findings indicated the possibility of designing computerized prescribing decision support that clinicians would accept its alert recommendation more. With more acceptance would come more widespread diffusion of these technologies, which would not only foster competition among its vendors to improve its features so that even more clinicians accept them and sales increase, but prices would also fall, making its diffusion even more widespread. This would help improve patient safety and the quality of healthcare delivery, and reduce health spending, again witness to the importance of competition and healthcare ICT in helping us achieve the dual objectives. Of course, other issues hinder the adoption of CPOE, in particular, and the major one, cost, applies to other healthcare ICT. Others include hospital variables for examples ownership, available resources, teaching status, and location. Thus, hospitals in rural and remote areas are less likely to adopt CPOE than those in urban settings, for-profit hospitals lag behind government and not-for-profit hospitals, and teaching hospitals, with more beds and nurse-to-bed staffing proportions, more than non-teaching ones. That research showed that medical technology adoption for example of ultrasound machines and computed tomography (CT) scanners) is higher greater among for-profit than not-for profit hospitals suggests that for-profit hospitals tend to adopt strategic healthcare ICT than do not-for-profit hospitals, which brings not only competitive issues but those regarding qualms about returns on investments (ROI) squarely to the fore[12, 13]. How do such issues influence healthcare ICT adoption in publicly funded health systems? Is there disconnect between the direction of the paradigm shift in healthcare delivery and the conceptualization of healthcare delivery by for-profit healthcare providers? What are the cost ramifications of this disconnect for the overall health system? Indeed, how strategic are these investment decisions in a healthcare milieu in flux? How would, for example, continuing efforts to unravel the mechanisms of contemporary healthcare delivery within the context of the consumer-focused healthcare model, with competitive forces and healthcare ICT playing key roles in achieving the dual objectives play out in this regard? There is no doubt for example about the need to secure the prerogative of the healthcare consumer in his/her health matters because premium differences, adjusted for risk, reflect the total annual per capita cost. As we have noted in this discussion, the choices of the healthcare consumer would likely be financially discerning if knowing he/she had a financial stake in the choices of health plans for example, which would exert market pressure on healthcare delivery systems to be inventive in reducing total healthcare cost. Would the service offering mix of hospitals not in fact need reviewing as part of this inventiveness for example, with the initiation of services tailored to the needs of the areas they serve, including preventive programs? Would this not require healthcare providers also to consider focusing on their core competences or targeting market niches? Are these competitive forces not eventually going to require an equally discerning approach to investments in technologies, including healthcare ICT, and would this not increase the chances of the realization of the technologies' ROI? A recent research study published in the Jan/Feb 2006 issue of Health Affairs noted for example that consumer-driven plans result in lower costs and increased use of preventive and chronic care services, but the researcher cautioned that these findings are preliminary. The researchers also noted that tax-advantaged accounts paired with high-deductibles would likely increase pressure on hospitals for more price transparency and pricing uniformity, and could reduce hospital spending by reducing use. These are the central issues we have touched on in our discussion thus far, and in support of which there is likely to be even more research evidence in the days ahead. Again, as evident in our discussion, it is not only critical to rectify the information asymmetry in the health industry for us to continue to see the benefits of consumer-focused healthcare, we also need to facilitate information communication and sharing, for example, to make vital patient information available at the point of care (POC), for example. By making such information available as and when needed that would lead to more effective treatment we would be reducing morbidities and mortalities from illnesses significantly, which would reduce the need for hospitalizations, for example, and save substantial healthcare costs. No doubt, our expectations of our efforts to rectify information asymmetry must be realistic, as Herbert Simon (1916-

2001), the 1978 winner of the Nobel Memorial Prize in Economics, cautioned in his observations on the uncertainties that necessarily compromise decision-making in organizations, for examples regarding the future based on current information. In other words, we might never at any point in time have perfect and complete information for fully rational decision-making hence we must acknowledge our "bounded rationality," yet the more accurate and current information we have and provide to the healthcare consumer, the closer to rationality, the "satisficing," as Herbert termed deciding on the less optimal choice, would be. Should we therefore not do whatever we could to ensure the widespread implementation and use of the technologies, namely, healthcare ICT, that would enable us achieve our dual goals of improving healthcare delivery while also saving costs, from which hospitals would benefit too? There is no doubt that an ever increasing national health spending as a proportion of any country's Gross Domestic Product(GDP) is unsustainable, and that we cannot afford to tire seeking measures to close this increasing chasm between the increase in health expenditures and GDP. This would no doubt necessitate out-of-the-box approaches for examples regarding promoting healthcare ICT diffusion among all healthcare stakeholders, encouraging healthcare consumers to make choices that do not result in the worsening of the quality of care that they receive just because they want to be discerning and save money, this latter which might involve giving them more financial incentives. We also need to consider ways to encourage healthcare providers to buy and implement healthcare ICT, including incentives offered as part of their overall remuneration packages, and revisiting various remuneration models, for example, pay-for-performance, to determine and promote, which of them most meets the needs for helping to achieve the dual objectives mentioned earlier. Organizations such as the AHRQ are helping in this regard. For example, it recently developed a pay-for-performance (P4P) tool, Pay for Performance: A Decision Guide for Purchasers, to assist employers, health plans, Medicaid agencies, and others planning to commence a pay-for-performance program. The tool would facilitate decision-making regarding designing, implementing, and assessing the activity. AHRQ Director Carolyn M. Clancy, M.D., announced the development of the tool in a speech to the Georgetown University Hospital professional staff on May 4, 2006. The decision guide poses 20 key questions that leaders from employer groups, health plans, or other health care purchasing groups ought to ask themselves as they muse over adopting the P4P program. The tool has questions such as if to partner with other organizations, focus on clinicians or hospitals first, mandate provider participation or leave them as voluntary; financial resource allocation, and addressing provider concerns regarding risk adjustment for illness severity, each question followed by a discussion on likely options and potential inadvertent consequences. It also has special advice for Medicaid agencies and Medicaid managed care plans. With regard encouraging doctors to implement healthcare ICT, in Alberta, Canada, almost 3000 physicians have benefited from the Physician Office System Program (POSP), a government incentive to encourage office automation. The 5-year-old incentive program, its costs at about $70 million so far, offers physicians as much as $35 520 in monthly installments over 4 years, intended to cover 70% of the cost of hardware, software and networking, the doctors expected to pay the remaining 30%. About 53% of the province s practicing physicians have implemented healthcare ICT, the highest rate in Canada, of which, over 80% are currently utilizing or switching to electronic medical records (EMR). Does this not attest to the benefits of such incentive programs in promoting healthcare ICT diffusion? According to the Alberta Medical Association, doctors forfeited about 1.5% in fee increases during contract talks in 2001 to assign money to the program. Some would argue that Alberta doctors, working in an Oil-rich province, and who successfully negotiated a 22% wages increase over 2 years in 2001, could afford to forfeit part of this wage. Others would counter that but they did so voluntarily, which is testimony to the power of persuasion in effecting attitudinal changes, and of that of intersectoral collaboration among government officials and healthcare professionals among others in our efforts to promote healthcare ICT diffusion. The program s components include vendor conformance and usability requirements, with doctors required to choose VCUR-certified products in order to receive funding. Change management is also a key aspect of the program, a network of private sector resources and physician mentors providing these services.

There is also the Privacy Impact Assessment that mandates doctors to inform the province s Information and Privacy Commissioner formally on their plans to protect patient information. Should other provinces in Canada, and indeed, other healthcare jurisdictions not adopt the Alberta or a similar approach to promoting healthcare ICT diffusion? Considering the immense benefits of healthcare ICT in reducing medical errors for which there is research evidence as noted earlier, should we not focus on devising other, novel approaches to promoting the widespread implementation of these technologies? Should we, indeed not be exploring ways to enhance the interaction of the tripartite subsystems mentioned earlier, which as we have seen are crucial to our achieving our dual objectives of delivering qualitative healthcare cost-effectively? To recap the theoretical postulates we have advanced in our discussion, competition is necessary for our survival, which latter is our natural tendency. Our physiology is on the go, hence our natural state is a driven state, the drive, propelling us forward to interact and transact with others. Is it therefore surprising that diseases ravage us when we are sedentary, and does activity not strengthen us and improve our health and well-being? Our language has made us superior to other living beings in this regard. It is the vessel for information acquisition, storage, and transmission, and information is the essential constituent of our transactions, hence the source of our competitive edge. What is more, it has helped us develop the technologies that facilitate the transmission of information in our transactions, including the processes involved in healthcare delivery. Processes incur costs and occur in time, which latter being in constant motion, therefore require measuring and pricing. By facilitating processes, these technologies therefore reduce costs. Should we therefore, ensure that we use these technologies to promote competition, hence improve the quality of healthcare delivery, and simultaneously reduce healthcare costs? Few would likely disagree with an affirmative answer to this all-embracing question.

References

1. L.M. Nichols et al., "Are Market Forces Strong Enough to Deliver Efficient Health Care Systems? Confidence Is Waning," *Health Affairs* 23, no. 2 (2004): 8-21.

2. V.R. Fuchs, "The 'Competition Revolution' in Health Care," *Health Affairs 7,* no. 3 (1988): 5-24.

3. Available at: http://www.conferenceboard.ca/press/documents/futurehealth.pdf
Accessed on May 06, 2006

4. Available at:
http://www3.who.int/whosis/country/compare.cfm?country=GBR&indicator=PcTot
EOHinIntD&language=english
Accessed on May 07, 2006

5. McGrail K, Green B, Barer ML, Evans RG, Hertzman C, Normand C. Age, costs of acute and long-term care and proximity to death: evidence for 1987-88 and 1994-95 in British Columbia. *Age and Ageing* 2000; 29:249-53

6. Barer ML, Evans RG, Hertzman C. Avalanche, or glacier? Health care and the demographic rhetoric. *Canadian Journal on Aging* 1995; 14(2):193-224.

7. Demers M. Factors explaining the increase in cost for physician care in Quebec's elderly population. *Canadian Medical Association Journal* 1996; 155(11):1555-60.

8. Department of Health, "Open and Staffed Critical Care Beds at 13 January 2005," Form KH03a, 11 March 2005, www.performance.doh.gov.uk/
Accessed on May 08, 2006

9. Department of Health, "Publication of Latest Statistics on Bed Availability and Occupancy for England 2000‾01," Press Release (London: Department of Health, 19 September 2001).

10. Available at: http://www.usatoday.com/money/industries/health/2006-05-09-shop-side_x.htm
Accessed on May 09, 2006

11. Shah NR, Seger AC, Seger DL, et al. Improving acceptance of computerized prescribing alerts in ambulatory care. J Am Med Inform Assoc 2006 Jan-Feb; 13(1):5-11.

12. Wang BB. et al., "Factors Influencing Health Information System Adoption in American Hospitals," *Health Care Management* Review 30, no. 1 (2005): 44-51.

13. Birkmeyer CM. et al.,"Will Electronic Order Entry Reduce Health Care Costs?" *Effective Clinical Practice 5,* no. 2 (2002): 67

ICT and Healthcare Costs

The increasing gap between the projected expenditures on health services provision

for the elderly and disabled and the revenues to fund these services constitute perhaps
the most significant challenge that health systems in the developed world would
confront in the years ahead. The need to act to prevent the overwhelming of Medicare
in the U.S. for example and health systems in general across the developed world by
the anticipated surge in healthcare utilization, as baby-boomers turn seniors in about
five years, becomes even more urgent that with population aging would be reduction
in the number of active workers to fund health services. Experts in health and relat ed
fields have been examining diverse scenarios for healthcare service provision for the
elderly and related issues of concern. Dana Goldman and his associates at RAND for
example, used a detailed microsimulation model called the Future Elderly Model
(FEM) 1. This model essentially simulates changes in health status of the elderly,
including deaths, over a year from estimated service usage based on current health
status. Incorporating new seniors yearly, the researchers were able to predict medical
costs and health status way ahead. One of the conclusions these and some other
researchers reached was the increased health spending technological innovation of

uncertain cost-effectiveness would engender. However, should this necessarily be so? Does it not depend on the technologies in question? Do the technologies that we use not depend on the orientation of our health services? Could not implement healthcare ICT whose overall benefits would outweigh their aggregate costs, even were they some of the most expensive? Witness the costs of equipping hospitals with expensive medical technologies that people use for services that other less expensive technologies could diagnose, or the need to use which they could prevent in the first place. Should we not be factoring the paradigm shift in healthcare delivery toward population health with the increasing conceptualization of healthcare along primary, secondary, and tertiary prevention in our projections on the future of health services provision for our seniors, and indeed, everyone else? Should we also not be examining this paradigm shift as backed by strategic intent rooted in our appreciation of the finiteness of our resources? A recent survey of Quebec s ERs by Gesca, a Quebec newspaper chain revealed that wait times in Montreal are significantly longer that in other parts of the province. For example, for an ER bed, Hotel-Dieu Hospital in downtown Montreal had a 28.2 hour-average wait time versus 15.9 hours outside the city. The question would be why this is so. Some of course would no doubt say it is the pressure on health services by more people living in the metropolis, but would the fewer numbers of doctors working outside cities not counter this position? Are people living in the city less healthy, or are they using health services more needlessly just because the services are there? Could one conclude therefore that medical technologies, which doubtless are also more prevalent in the cities, must inevitably, drive healthcare costs sky-high, even just in the cities, such as in Montreal, not to mention the entire province? In other words, could we not find and replicate in Montreal, whatever the reasons are, if possible, for the shorter wait times outside the city, and if not develop unique solutions for it to reduce wait times? In the U.S, a new report also highlighted the sometimes-significant variations in Medicare spending on beneficiaries with chronic illnesses, in different states and hospitals, although the increased spending does not result in longer life for beneficiaries or higher satisfaction with their quality of care. According to a May 16, 2006 *USAToday* report, the study, by the Dartmouth Atlas Project, looked at records of hospital care, tests and physician visits provided to 4.7 million Medicare beneficiaries in the last two years of their lives, participants aged 67 years and older, had at least one of 12 chronic illnesses, and passed away between 2000 and 2003. The study showed that Medicare's highest spending averagely $39,810, was for participants in New Jersey, the District of Columbia, California and New York, in decreasing order, the least, averagely, $23,697, for those in Idaho, Iowa, West Virginia and North Dakota, also in decreasing order. Do these figures ring true, vis-à-vis the Quebec wait lists figures mentioned above, and are there common factors operational, for example, population density, differential health status, and service overuse? This study indeed, also found that the New Jersey participants had the highest average number of physician visits during the last six months of their lives, 41.5, compared to the lowest, in Utah, at 17. Hawaii participants spent most days in hospital, the average number of days in the hospital during the same period, 16.4, which for Utah with the lowest average were 7.3. Paradoxically, participants that received the most care for each chronic illness had the highest mortality rates, according to the study. The study's findings on hospital utilization by the participants are instructive. During the period that the study examined, hospitalization and ICU admission rates were five times higher at some major academic hospitals than at others, the former highest for participants at New York State University Medical Center (NYUMC), an average of 32.1 days, versus 12.9 days for participants at the Mayo Clinic facility, St. Mary's Hospital. For ICU admission, participants at the University of California-Los Angeles Medical Center spent an average of 11.4 days, versus 3.3 days for those at UC-San Francisco Medical Center. Medicare expenditures also varied by hospital with an average of $79,280 for services during the last two years of the participants' lives, at NYUMC, versus $37,271, for those at the Mayo Clinic. Do these figures reflect a flawed pattern of decision-making regarding care? Are these seniors receiving care that they do not need, for example, expensive investigations, and specialist consultations, and could they have fared just as well receiving less expensive care albeit with a different focus, in ambulatory/community/ and domiciliary settings? Do we not need to examine this study closely and act on the possible reasons for its intriguing findings? Are these findings pointers to some of the explanations to those of the RAND study mentioned earlier, for example, on the increases in healthcare spending the study found medical technologies would engender in the future, and is this not time we took aversive action on such developments? There is no doubt that the number of seniors in the U.S and other developed countries, and indeed, in many other countries in the developing world would increase over time. Figures released by the Kaiser Family Foundation on May 18, 2006 indicate that for 2004, the numbers of retail prescription drugs filled at pharmacies (per Capita by Age) were 4.2, 10.4, and 25.5, for the age groups, 0-18 years, 19-64 years, and 65 years and above, respectively, the figure for seniors is about twice for the two other groups combined. To be sure, U.S drug expenditures grew 8.2% in 2004, less than half the growth rate five years ago. Health care spending increased 7.9% to $1.9 trillion in 2004, $6,280 per person, or 16% of the country's Gross Domestic Product (GDP), about as much as in 2003. Overall, health-spending rate slowed relative to 2000-2002 for both public and private payers, 30% of the combined increase between 2002 and 2004, prescription drugs making up 11% of this spending, although not as much as its share of the increase in recent years and substantially slower in unqualified terms2. However, with the expected increase in the numbers of seniors, would these figures not even be higher, particularly if we did nothing to rationalize resource utilization? The health sector's percentage of the GDP increased only 0.1% in 2004, due partly to an above-average economic growth rate, 70% during the same year versus 4.8% the previous year. Nonetheless, what would healthcare spending be like in particular, in the U.S and other developed countries, with access to sophisticated medical technologies with seniors, and indeed, others, receiving treatment that they hardly need and would make little if any difference to their chronic illnesses? Would this not in fact adversely affect economic growth rates in these countries? Should we not pursue a different paradigm of care for the seniors that would still deliver qualitative health services, but which they need, and at less costs? What role could the more widespread implementation of healthcare ICT play in the achievement of these dual objectives? We noted above that health spending slowed in the U.S in 2004, but private payers were essentially responsible for more of this slowing than public payers, with spending by the former down to 7.6% compared to 8.6% in 2003. Out-of-pocket spending increased by 5.5% in 2004, that is, a lesser portion of overall and private health spending. Public health spending on the other hand increased by 8.2%, 47% of aggregate growth in 2004, versus 43% in 2003. Private health insurance premiums slowed in 2004, and benefits remained steady, with decreasing drug spending buffering increased hospital and physician spending increases. Here again, we see the possible consequences of not optimizing resources, for examples in the interplay of the use/misuse/or even abuse of hospitalization, prescription medications, and expensive investigations and procedures. Could spending on prescription medications be falling because of increased use of the often-cheaper but just as effective, generics over brand medications? With private payer contribution to health spending falling, and assuming it continues to do so, for how long could Medicare continue to afford to pay the ever-increasing bill, which increased 8.9% to $309 billion in 2004, compared to its 6.6% increase in 2003 it would then receive due, for example to unnecessary hospitalizations? Is this why some insist that cost sharing some way or another is necessary for any health system to survive? The Medicare Prescription Drug, Improvement, and Modernization Act (MMA) of 2003 that increased payments for capitated health plans and rural providers no doubt played a role in Medicare's higher spending in 2004, and the Part D drug benefit plan would perhaps play an even greater role from 2006. Could we prevent the effect of the latter for example by providing seniors with the necessary information to make the right treatment, including medication choices, in consultation with their doctors? Could healthcare ICT not help in providing them with such information, via the concept of targeted health information dissemination? Is this not quite urgent considering the significant increases in Medicare attributed to home health and physician spending in 2004, due to increased service usage, under the prospective payment system (PPS), with growth in spending for physician services ($8 billion) accounting for almost 35% (23% in 2003) of the increase in personal health care (PHC) spending by Medicare? Medicare spending on home health services increased

19% in 2004, significantly over previous years, and might continue to increase without proactive action based on an understanding of the issues involved in these increases. The increase in home services in particular demands exploration. There is no doubt about the desirability of ambulatory/community/domiciliary health service provision for our seniors, being responsible for most of these services but could we not provide them more cost-effectively, while still assuring there quality? Again, are we emphasizing the wrong types of home services, overusing resources, or even abusing them? How could healthcare ICT help in this regard? Funding is another important issue. For example, Medicare funds them via general revenue taxes, which would likely increase the more the health spending, with funds from payrolls taxes and premiums, which funded 79% of Medicare spending in 1979, down to 63% in 2004, while funds via general revenue taxes increased from 21% to 35% during the same period. Could the public afford to keep enduring a perpetual increase in taxes, or have part B services compromised by health spending guzzling a disproportionate chunk of the services general revenue taxes fund? Should these considerations not inspire the public to take measures to prevent this scenario, for example to embrace healthcare ICT-based disease prevention and treatment measures, and more-rational use of health services, particularly hospitalization, and costly medical technologies? Commenting on the Dartmouth Atlas Project data mentioned earlier, Elliott Fisher, a professor of medicine at Dartmouth noted, "These data allow patients, purchasers (such as insurers and Medicare) and policy makers to see what's happening to patients with chronic illness," adding that the differences between hospitals have " huge implications for what patients pay in terms of their co-payments. "These differences could also have important ramifications for the overall quality of healthcare delivery, not just in countries that have predominantly-privately funded health systems but also in those with public funding. Imaging paying for unnecessary services or healthcare resources becoming depleted as a result in public funded health systems such as in Canada, and the U.K. Could this not result, ultimately in lesser quality services and/or possible tax increases in both instances, and indeed, in any health system? There is no doubt that this is a key area for urgent consideration in any health system.

Providing qualitative health services is desirable for any age group, and for any

disease condition, but wasting healthcare resources is not, and in fact, is harmful not only to a country's economy, but also to its ability to provide these services in the long term. We certainly need to start taking a critical look at all the issues involved in the soaring healthcare costs in contemporary times, and find ways by which we could stem this tide, literally, and still provide our seniors, and everyone else the qualitative healthcare that they need, and not that they wish, or which someone taking decisions for them does. The latter point underscores the need for every stakeholder, doctor, patient, relative, and others, to have the right information, at the right time, and of course use this information in decision making on health issues. Information asymmetry in the health industry is pervasive, and persistent, and needs urgent attention to rectify it. Progress in medical knowledge continues apace, and bears significantly on our understanding of health and illness. We all need to know about these developments, and those that interest and have relevance for us and our loved ones, or others we know. The concept of targeted health information dissemination is one that could facilitate this knowledge, and healthcare ICT is crucial in helping us achieve this goal. Is it any wonder that a U.S. National Institutes of Health (NIH) independent panel to evaluate the available evidence on the safety and effectiveness of multivitamin/minerals (MVMs) has recommended a more informed approach to the use of multivitamin/mineral for chronic disease prevention? The panel, which released a draft statement of its findings on May 17, 2006, after two days of expert presentations, public discussion, and panel deliberations, advised on certain specific supplements and on the need for more rigorous scientific research before making strong recommendations on the use of MVM to prevent chronic diseases. The panel's findings concern the healthy and excluded pregnant women, children, or individuals with disease. According to J. Michael McGinnis, M.D., M.P.P., Senior Scholar with the Institute of Medicine of the National Academy of Sciences and panel chair, "Half of American adults are taking MVMs and the bottom line is that we don t know for sure that they re benefiting from them. In fact, we re concerned that some people may be getting too much of certain nutrients. These are of course legitimate concerns not just in terms of the consumer pouring money down the drain due to an expectation/benefit mismatch, but also because of the possible adverse consequences of some of these products on health used for example, in excess. Does this not call for the public having accurate and current information on them, but how do people obtain such information? Should we not deliver the information to them via cost-effective, and efficient, healthcare ICT-backed targeted health information dissemination? Are they likelier or not to receive unbiased and current health information this way? The panel made certain specific recommendations, for example, the combined use of calcium and vitamin D supplementation for postmenopausal women to protect bone health, and advised non-smoking adults with early-stage, age-related macular degeneration, a possible cause of blindness, use anti-oxidants and zinc. It also reiterated an earlier, Centers for Disease Control and Prevention (CDC) counsel that women of childbearing age take daily folate to prevent their infants developing birth defects of the brain and spinal cord. It did not find compelling evidence to recommend beta-carotene supplements, some sort of vitamin A, for the public, but did to warn smokers against using them due to the association of regular use by smokers of the vitamin to an increase prevalence of lung cancer. The panel could not conclude either way on the value of the use of MVMs to prevent chronic diseases, noting that most people that use them for this purpose also practice healthy lifestyles such as eating right and exercising, which makes it difficult to ascribe the benefits to health specifically to the MVMs. The panel noted the risks involved with using MVMs, for example, adverse effects due to their excessive use, which could occur relatively readily coupled with consumption of fortified foods, and the use of large doses of single vitamins and minerals. These safety concerns apparently prompted the panel to recommend that the Food and Drug Administration (FDA) amend the regulation of dietary supplements, including MVMs, and indeed that the

U.S Congress broadens FDA's power and resources to mandate those that manufacture these products to disclose adverse events, to assure quality, and to include reporting information on dietary supplement labels. The latter would make it easier for the consumer to report these events. The panel also made a number of specific recommendations on future researches that would make them more rigorous, and their findings more valid, hence safer to recommend to the public. Would the public not in fact be better able to make equally valid judgments regarding disbursing their funds on these products, and their expectations of their benefits? Would such more rational health decisions not on the aggregate help improve the health of the people and reduce health spending? Consider the following recent development regarding cancer of the cervix, the second commonest cancer women have. An FDA advisory panel, the Vaccine and Related Biological Products Advisory Committee, on May 18, 2006 voted unanimously for FDA to approve a vaccine that blocks viruses that cause most cervical cancer. The panel concurred that that the vaccine, Gardasil, which Merck and Co. makes is safe and effective, and according to the firm could reduce the prevalence of deaths worldwide from cervical cancer by over 75%. The vaccine would cost between $300 and $500 given in three shots over three months, which some consider pricey, but no doubt, many would consider taking the shots a rational decision. The vaccine protects against the two forms of human papillomavirus (HPV) thought to cause about 70% of cervical cancer, and against two others responsible for 90% of genital warts, all four transmitted via sexual intercourse. The FDA would decide on June 08, 2006 on the panel's recommendation, which they typically accept. Half of sexually active adults have HPV, the cause of cervical cancers responsible for the deaths annually of approximately 290,000 women worldwide, 3,500 of them in the U.S. Regular Pap smear screening could detect precancerous lesions and early cancer, and with this new vaccine, things have just gotten much better regarding our efforts to eliminate cancer of the cervix. "Gardasil has the potential to meet an unmet medical need as the first vaccine to prevent cervical cancer," Merck's Dr. Patrick Brill-Edwards told the advisory committee. Many experts agree but cautioned that the vaccine should complement, and not replace Pap smear screening, to which Merck agreed, a very critical point to note when passing this information on to women. Indeed, according to Amy Allina, program director of the National Women's Health Network, "We would like to see the FDA mandate some sort of labeling or other mechanism to communicate to health care providers and patients the continued need for regular cervical screening. " Merck has indicated that females aged 9 years to 26 years, could use the vaccine but is best before females start to have sex. It is possible that the National Advisory Committee on Immunization Practices would recommend routine vaccination with the vaccine once FDA approves it in June 2006. Some worry that the vaccine would promote sexual activity among youths, but we cannot ignore its effect of reducing cancer rates and must continue our sex education efforts as there are still many diseases such as HIV out there for which sexual indiscretion puts one at risk. It is also important to note that Gardasil does not automatically protect against the viruses in persons already infected, and could actually increase their risk for developing precursors to cervical cancer. It does not also protect against other viruses, and in five cases of women who got the shots about the time of conception, they had children with birth defects. Merck also tested the vaccine in boys. However, it has not reported on their recommendations on the vaccine for males. There is no doubt about the need to deliver this information to parents and to young people now, and as soon as FDA approves the vaccine, and policy decision taken on whether or not to give it routinely to young girls. There is also need to encourage further research into vaccine development for other viruses. We might be reducing health spending significantly overall and in the long term by so doing, not to mention the burden of disease on individuals that have cancer of the cervix, their families, and on society. Persistent and interdisciplinary genomic research efforts since 1990, for example has now yielded full dividend considering the recent announcement in mid-May 2006 of the sequencing of the last chromosome in the Human Genome, which has an estimated 20,000 to 25,000 genes strewn literally on chromosomes found within the nucleus of a cell. Associated with about 350 illnesses including cancer, Alzheimer's and Parkinson's disease, Chromosome 1, has almost twice as many genes, 3,141, as the average chromosome, and constitutes 8% of the human genetic code. According to Dr Simon Gregory, head of the sequencing project at the Sanger Institute in England, "this achievement effectively closes the book on an important volume of the Human Genome Project. Chromosome 1 "is the region of the genome to which the greatest number of diseases has been localized," he added, being the largest and with most genes. Published online in *Nature*, its sequencing took a team of 150 British and American scientists 10 years to finish, but the efforts are no doubt worth the while. Researchers worldwide now have a veritable database from which to mine valuable information that would assist in improving the diagnosis and treatment of such diseases as cancers, autism, mental disorders and many more. Furthermore, the sequencing of chromosome 1 has resulted in the identification of over 1,000 new genes, and Gregory also noted, "We are moving into the next phase which will be working out what the genes do and how they interact," and of the processes that cause genetic diversity in populations. Indeed, chromosome 1 s genetic map has resulted in the discovery of a gene for a common form of cleft lip and palate. The researchers also identified 4,500 new single nucleotide polymorphisms (SNPs), the variations in human DNA responsible for individual uniqueness, and that contain clues regarding why some people are prone to diseases such as cancer or malaria, how best to diagnose and treat them, and their response to treatment and the probable outcome of the condition. Should there not be more research funds invested in unraveling the secrets locked in this and other chromosomes and could we not derive valuable knowledge thereof? Would such knowledge not help us reduce the prevalence of many diseases, some of which are more prevalent among our seniors, and could this not help improve the quality of life or our seniors, reduce hospitalization rates, and the use of costly prescription drugs, thus overall health spending? There is no doubt about the need for a broad-based conceptualization of the issues involved in looking ahead at healthcare delivery to our seniors, within the context of the more general challenges confronting our health systems. Research promotion as an important aspect of this all-inclusive perspective should not only be interdisciplinary, and intersectoral, it should involve collaboration between the private and public sectors, both within a country, and between countries. The success of such efforts, as the example of the genome sequencing mentioned above illustrates often depends on the knowledge and expertise of many coalescing. Because of the substantial costs sometimes involved, such collaboration also spreads out the cost, making it easier for the individual partners to bear. Furthermore, this sort of collaboration also underscores the multifaceted roles of healthcare ICT in our health quality improvement and cost containment efforts-mix, as these technologies would be crucial to facilitating communication and information sharing among geographically dispersed research associates.

Whichever way we look at it, resources are finite, and require prudent management

to optimize. Ignoring this principle is courting escalation in health spending, which could only further drain dwindling resources. Thirty years ago, in the U.S., certificate of need programs, some form of "regionalization," characterized by a purposeful effort at resource optimization, with a rational and efficient distribution of specialized procedures such as coronary artery bypass graft (CABG) surgery and percut aneous coronary intervention (PCI) based on specified criteria, for example, population and geography, were rife. The goal, to limit spending on health services, in particular on expensive interventional cardiovascular procedures, and technologies3. These certificates, however, are essentially all gone, cancelled in 19 states in its entirety, for CABG in 25, but did these certificates help improve healthcare quality or reduce costs, and should we revisit them considering the anticipated further increase in the already-high healthcare spending in the U.S and many developed countries? A recent article published in vol. 295, pp2141-7, 2006 of the Journal of the American Medical Association examined these issues. Researchers explored the link between certificates of need and treatment of a medical condition, acute myocardial infarction (AMI), not controlled by such certificates, although often involves the use of procedures that the certificates control, namely, CABG surgery and PCI, jointly termed coronary revascularization procedures. They noted the less likelihood of hospitalizations for coronary revascularization, for Medicare patients with AMI in states with certificates of need, the reverse true for those without. The former were also less likely to undergo revascularization at the admitting hospital, however, more so at a transfer hospital, although the overall effect was that they were less likely to undergo revascularization within the first 2 days. Furthermore, despite the lower early revascularization rates, there was no difference in the risk-adjusted 30-day mortality between the two groups of patients. What are the implications of these findings for regionalizing AMI care, while ensuring strict adherence to the specific guidelines for the care of such patients? Would such regionalization result in cost savings without compromising the quality of care delivery[5]? Should we also have designated ST-segment-elevation myocardial infarction (STEMI) centers, for patients with this diagnosis for who evidence suggests could benefit most with early access to PCI [6]? The answers to such questions would no doubt help us better optimize the use of our hospitals and develop the appropriate services for example, equipping ambulances able to perform 12-lead electrocardiograms, and to train paramedics on appropriate actions to take, for example to transport patients with STEMI to STEMI centers. Others include establishing prehospital triage protocols for patients with STEMI based for example on geographical constraints or otherwise to access to PCI hospitals and STEMI centers, ensuring minimal delay in accessing these required services. We are going to need to develop the appropriate criteria for regionalizing care for AMI in future, including ensuring appropriate geographical distribution, attention to disease distribution, and demographic characteristics, and indeed, we need to start to examine these issues as many more become seniors over time. It is important to set the right parameters based on the above and other considerations rather than arbitrarily, since for example research has shown that designating too many STEMI centers whimsically or based on pressure from interest groups could result in worse outcomes if the centers did fewer procedures. In other words, as the study mentioned above shows, there is a direct link between volume and outcome for PCI in AMI patients, with centers that do more having better outcomes[7]. Would such careful planning of these services not help save costs and still deliver qualitative care to these patients? Should we not re-examine some procedures and start implementing them.

For example, the use of aspirin and [beta]-blockers at the times of hospital admission and discharge result in better outcomes that we need to incorporate it in standard practice and measure for quality evaluation as we do other major process measures such as time from arrival at the hospital and delivery of fibrinolytic therapy (door-to-needle time). Others are time from arrival to PCI (door-to-balloon time) procedures and measure interhospital process differences to benchmark quality services and improve those centers necessary to upgrade. Based on the findings of this study, regionalization seems to have the potential to deliver qualitative healthcare and save costs. Should we apply its principles to other diseases, and service offerings? Quebec province in Canada has a "complementarity" plan that proposes the reshuffling of medical services as a cost-cutting measure, for example, transferring complex cardiac surgery and other specializations to specific facilities that would promote resource optimization hence deliver higher quality services, and save costs, although the plan faces stiff opposition among healthcare professionals, and some of the hospitals involved. The concept of "centers of excellence" is another closely related option, which both the private and public sectors could explore. This involves establishing and staffing tertiary centers for the treatment of specific conditions, again, the distribution of these centers based on determined parameters, and could in fact involve interstate and interprovincial collaboration to serve individuals living near state and provincial borders. Strategically located, such centers would serve as apical referral centers, obviating the need to duplicate services, some, where their underutilization could only escalate healthcare costs. Such centers as noted earlier could be private enterprises, and in publicly funded health systems such as in Canada, established by provincial/territorial governments, and not under any particular health region, more so if interprovincial. Hospitals already exist in many Canadian provinces that serve special needs of the entire province, which could form the foundation for these centers of excellence. Just as it is not practical to build a hospital in every town or settlement, recognizing the need to rationalize their establishment vis-à-vis the services that they offer is also just being realistic, a necessary position considering increasing healthcare costs. Increasing healthcare costs indeed, prompted the concern of U.S. former Federal Reserve Chair Greenspan in a speech to the Bond Market Association on May 19, 2006, about the escalating costs of Medicare, which he described as unsustainable, and noted could ultimately cause the U.S federal debt to increase and interest rates too, and significantly. Indeed, every payer, regardless of a health system's funding model, is feeling the pinch, literally of these increasing healthcare costs. Their effects on private firms have been devastating for both the companies, with regressing profits, and their employees, with the recent massive layoffs by Ford Motor Co. and General Motors. Indeed, they are going to have profound ramifications for the future of healthcare for the increasing numbers of individuals that would retire from these companies and turn seniors in the near future. Even the Japanese companies, which adopted an essentially different approach to their employees' health benefits, will soon have to deal with the benefits' issues in the U.S when some of their employees, many recruited in the mid-1980s and still working, start to retire in the next few years. Toyota's American division, for example, has only 258 retired production workers, compared to General Motors' over 400,000 retirees. However, in 2011 and 2012, 1,700 of Toyota's employees will be eligible for retirement, roughly 6% of its current labor force. However, unlike their contemporaries in the General Motors (GM), Ford, and Chrysler, they will be responsible for much more of the costs and the risks of retirement. In addition to a monthly $50/service year paycheck up to $1,500 maximum, which accrues after 30 years of service, an average GM retiree with 30 years service receives a supplement with their monthly check as high as $3,000 until they are 62 years old. Furthermore, until 2005, when GM and the United Automobile Workers Union (UAW) agreed on a deal for retirees to cover co-pays and deductibles, the company funds their healthcare costs. With an unfunded liability of $85 billion (current money) to cover future health care costs for workers and retirees, almost eight times the market value of the entire firm, GM, understandably could ill-afford generous health benefits and soaring healthcare costs. Incidentally, with the burden of such costs per vehicle at $1,500, $1,400, and $1,100, for General Motors, Chrysler, and Ford, in the U.S., does the consumer not share part of these companies' healthcare costs? Even their pension plans guzzle enough money to create serious concern for them, and would it not with GM for example since 1992 investing in them, $56 billion in stock and cash, which the company, in a bid to reduce, offered all its 105,000 U.A.W. employees buyout packages up to $140,000. Government in Japan covers retirees' healthcare and funds more of workers' pensions, but in the U.S. Toyota not only pays part of its retirees' healthcare costs, albeit much less in the same year for example, than GM's $5.4 billion in 2005. It would also pay about $700 million in pension benefits in FY2006, ended in March, even if less than one tenth of GM's in the same period. It is not only Toyota that is not offering its workers free health and defined pension checks, certain accompaniments of retirement package deals between the unions and the major U.S firms post WWII, under which "legacy" strain the major U.S auto companies now labor, is why even they are no longer paying their retirees' healthcare costs in full. As with the Japanese companies that require their retirees to pay part of their healthcare premiums predicated on years of service, GM, and other U.S firms now also do. Besides Honda, none of the other major Japanese auto firms in the U.S offers a defined-benefit pension, hence a monthly check for retirees, and in general all exclude them from the company health plan on being 65 years old, given money in lieu that they could use to purchase added insurance to Medicare. With retirees and their dependents outnumbering present-day workforce of GM by a ratio of 3:1, is it any wonder that G.M. abolished health care coverage for its salaried, nonunion retirees hired post-1993, for example, and in 2006 stopped their defined-contribution pension plan? These issues would likely have adverse implications for healthcare coverage for seniors in the years ahead, particularly considering the open secret that baby boomers, for example, have not been very diligent about saving for retirement, which nonetheless, their assets, particularly real estate, which have appreciated in value in many cases recently, would likely cushion. Indeed, many seniors are already tapping the equity on their homes, for example via reverse mortgage loans even with their high upfront costs and limited payouts, to fund their retirements as their traditional income sources, such as Social Security benefits, pensions, savings and part-time work are proving undependable, as the above analysis shows. Do these issues not warrant a closer look therefore, on how we could reduce healthcare costs, for all payers, including individual seniors who as shown above are going to have to pay more of their healthcare costs with time? Put differently might seniors, and baby-boomers when they turn seniors possibly find health services unaffordable eventually, hence inaccessible, if healthcare costs continued to increase unchecked? Would it be unreasonable to deploy the appropriate healthcare ICT to facilitate the initiatives we have identified as needed to enable seniors to be able to afford and access healt h services that are demonstrably able to achieve these goals cost-effectively? Is a major part of the likelihood to succeed in reducing healthcare not a focus on this initiative-technology mix for the various healthcare conditions, and issues, peculiar to each country, and health jurisdiction? For example, and as we noted earlier, it makes intuitive sense not to invest in services that people do not need, and not to locate services where those that need them cannot access them. Designating services therefore involves a balancing act, but it is worth the efforts, considering the importance of rational resource allocation in cost containment, particularly as it offers quality improvement as well. Let us look at hospitalization costs again as they underscore this point. With increasingly longevity would likely come certain help problems, for example arthritis, with which would likely come the need for knee and hip replacement, and possibly that of other joints, among a variety of orthopedic problems such as fractures common in the elderly, and which invariably require the use of hospitals. Increasing demand and volume of procedures, increase in price, and the evolution of product mix based on medical progress and that of materials science and engineering, for examples, bio-implants, computer-assisted surgery, and minimally invasive surgery, not to mention the costs of the procedures, hospital stays, medications, and others are cost drivers for these procedures. In other words, we should be looking at the component processes of the final goal, for example, hip replacement, in order to have a more accurate picture of the costs involved in the exercise. Some of these costs are more obvious than others are, for example, that overweight and obesity are also cost drivers, as individuals with these problems tend to wear out their joints quicker. On the other hand, that the appliance manufacturer passes on the cost of having to look all over town and go through three sets of middlemen to find a machinist to work on a piece of cobalt chrome molybdenum required for the product might not be. Thus, just as it makes business sense for the manufacturer to be close to where the resources for production are, should we not be doing the same for these procedures rather than expecting to have an orthopedic surgeon in every hospital in every town? This brings us back to the various concepts of distributing hospital resources we mentioned earlier, such centers of excellence, where in fact, we could have "clusters" of professionals in related field serving specified geographical populations. This would no doubt help with the waist list problems in many publicly funded health systems as referrals would be better streamlined, particularly with peripheral doctors all hooked up to the electronic health records (EHR) systems serving that jurisdiction and via extensions, regionally, and nationally. In privately funded systems, such as in the U.S, it is even more likely that entrepreneurs and private healthcare providers would collaborate to establish such centers, taking into consideration a number of issues that would make their investments profitable while effectively delivery their service offerings.

Focalization of competencies either in the public or private healthcare system would

reduce operational costs in labor, supplies, and transportation, processes that indeed, healthcare ICT could help facilitate, for example, supply chain management software enabling the hospital to have real time contact with suppliers that could alert both parties to changing stock supplies, and storage and transportation hitches. Many hospitals invest in surgical equipments for examples that they do not use, because they do not have surgeons, say orthopedic surgeons. Would the resources invested in the theaters and on surgical supplies not be better used to collaborate with other jurisdictions to establish the service centers that would serve them all and cost-effectively. There is no doubt that each jurisdiction would need certain basic health services, again, the mix based on their unique needs, but as stated earlier, not every town needs to have every medical specialist. This is simply unrealistic. Thus, why should the jurisdiction invest in areas of Medical practice that they either do not need, or is not cost-effective to have in a particular town or city? Why should a border town X, in Canada for example with only a few thousand people purchase an MRI equipment, when there is a big city Y, two kilometers across the border that has one? Would it not be more cost effective for town X to outsource its MRI needs to city Y? Here is an example of the complexity of issues that today's health policy makers have to grapple with, and must, considering the tide of events, in particular, the increasing sophistication of the healthcare consumer's taste, in the context of skyrocketing healthcare costs. Thus, it would be necessary to tease out licensure issues between provinces and territories in Canada for instance, between which such outsourcing would mostly be occurring, and with the U.S governments, and indeed, others even in far-away countries such as India, where such outsourcing is already commonplace in the U.S. in fields such as Radiology. There are of course other issues such as remuneration, and incentives. This example also shows the need for increased attention to healthcare ICT issues by these countries. Outsourcing necessarily involves communication, across time zones, and between far-flung locations, which would be impossible without the necessary technological infrastructures, and the consensus on the standards to make them interoperable for examples. Yet, we could readily miss the opportunity to save significant healthcare costs not attending to these issues. Let us examine this issue a little further using the example of heart failure, a condition that about 5 million Americans have with 550,000 new cases diagnosed each year, and which costs the country an estimated $28 billion in associated healthcare costs annuallys. The condition is just as prevalent in many developed countries considering the increasing longevity in these countries. About 3% of all Canadians, aged 35 to 64 years have heart disease. Cardiovascular diseases (CVD) in general, are the leading causes of death in Canada and claim over 78,000 lives (about 36% of all deaths) in Canada each year. Many acute myocardial infarction (AMI) patients who survive their index hospitalization ultimately develop congestive heart failure (CHF), and hospitalized CHF patients fare even worse than AMI patients do, with a one-year mortality rate of 33%, even worse than most cancers, and over 30% of those who have heart disease are unable to work because of their illness. CVD also puts considerable and increasing economic strain on the country's health care system, estimated costs in 1998, approximately $19 billion, in $6.8 billion, and $11.6 billion direct and indirect costs, respectively, figures billed to increase with the population aging further. Indeed, with most of CHF patients for example, being seniors, should we therefore not expect more as the population ages and baby-boomers turn seniors in another five years, and the need for cardiac services to increase? There is no doubt that continuing efforts at reducing the high prevalence rate of the major risk factors such as dyslipidemias, diabetes, obesity, smoking, physical inactivity, and high blood pressure, would help reduce the epidemic of heart disease and stroke in Canada, and that healthcare ICT could help in the various campaign and other initiatives in this regard. We should also endeavor to understand the gender, age, geographical and other variations in these risk factors in other to design the best preventive and treatment programs for these heart diseases in general. These suggestions are applicable to other countries as well, particularly the developed countries where there are more similarities than differences in these variables, with programs that worked in one country, tried in another, and with continuous collaboration for exchange of ideas, and data that could help achieve the goals of reducing these risk factors. Such collaboration also underlines the need for health information technologies that could facilitate data and information sharing to be available and indeed, widespread. CHF has a 5-year mortality rate of 50%, most patients' health and quality of life in continual decline once diagnosed with the condition. However, recent clinical trials revealed that two types of implantable devices, the implantable cardioverter defibrillator (ICD) and the cardiac resynchronization therapy (CRT) devices, are beneficial to improve outcomes in patients with heart failure patients that have reduced left ventricular ejection fractions and left ventricular conduction anomalies. Indeed, their use is becoming commoner and indications broader, is cost-effective, and might eventually become standard practice for a wider variety of patients. Recent studies showed that, unlike before, patients receiving implantable cardioverter defibrillators, used to prevent sudden death related to cardiac arrhythmias for patients with a previous history of AMI and reduced left ventricular function by providing cardioversion in the event of life-threatening arrhythmias, need not to be refractory to medications and to undergo electrophysiological studies before eligibility for the implants[9]. Indeed, not only are the results of these studies making the use of these implants more widespread and standard practice, the Centers for Medicare & Medicaid Services (CMS) has expanded coverage for ICD implantation based on their findings. In other words, cardiac units lacking electrophysiological capabilities could now broaden the scope of their services to offer ICD implantation. It should therefore be possible for health regions in Canada, for example to establish strategically placed cardiac units in certain hospitals, even when they lack electrophysiologists. Recent studies also show the benefits of CRT devices, compared to customary pacemakers, which latter utilize leads that pace only the right side of the heart, resulting in left ventricular dyssynchrony, conduction delays, and eventually, heart failure. CRT on the other hand is able to coordinate the left- and right-sided heart contractions[10]. For patients that also need an ICD, both CRT and ICD devices are often combined (CRT-D), with recent studies showing that more patients would need and benefit from the insertion of these devices. Would health regions not save substantially focusing these services, including outsourcing them to private healthcare providers if this would facilitate access to care by some. Would it not be easier for such private healthcare providers even those whose cardiologists are not electrophysiologists, to undergo training in the Heart Rhythm Society (HRS) standardized clinical training guidelines for cardiologists that would enable them carry out these implantations, and then establish such services where they are lacking? Would this not complement available public health services, and make outsourcing by the former less expensive? Hospital CEOs need to revisit their cardiac service plans and decide whether broadening their service offering to include CRT and ICD treatment fits into their strategic plans, and if they had cardiac units, theirs too. This would help in deciding whether to provide these services in-house or to outsource them. They also need to define very clearly, the scope of the new service line and it should blend neatly into the establishment's mix of cardiac services to avoid disruption, and other adverse consequences of an outlier service. The decision should predicate on needs assessment, current and projected of targeted population, availability of in-house expertise, and of local competitive services, and of course a financial analysis of the effects of the projected revenue or savings from the proposed services versus current practice, and of course start-up and other costs, and training issues. These analyses would make decision making much easier, for example which hospital should provide the services, and whether they should outsource them, and if they currently refer patients to other hospitals within the public health system, to continue, or outsource the services to private healthcare providers. It is going to be increasingly important for hospital administrators and policy makers in publicly funded health systems such as in Canada and the U.K and indeed, all countries, to perform such analyses. This would help them to take appropriate decisions regarding translating crucial research findings into practical actions, which some studies indicate some health authorities do not as the following example shows. This study published in the march 2006 issue of the Journal of the American Geriatrics Society, looked at chronic heart failure (CHF) that randomized, controlled trials of posthospital CHF disease management have shown benefit patients and reduce costs, yet is not standard in the U.S[11]. The authors performed a literature review of 30 randomized, controlled trials of multidisciplinary outpatient CHF management, which in general resulted in improved patient outcomes. They found on e-mail survey of first authors that practices found effective in the U.S. studies in general did not continue or expand in 13 of 15 studies, in the main blamed on monetary constraints in 11 of 13, versus similar projects in other countries that often became enduring, as in 7 of 13. U.S. respondents mostly rated current quality of clinical care as good, those elsewhere, as excellent. The authors noted the differences in the model of CHF management implemented with recent Medicare reforms and those studied in health services research, the former, based on the model commercial disease-management firms use. They also recommended that policy-makers, health service researchers, and funding agencies develop more-effective methods for converting proven models of healthcare delivery into routine practice, and develop reforms to actualize the connections between research, policy, and practice. There is doubt about the soundness of this suggestion considering the implications of a recent study that found that heart failure patients hospitalized in the U.S are less likely to expire in the first month after discharge than are those hospitalized in Canada, mortality rates, 8.9% vs. 10.7%. The study compared the 30-day and 1-year outcomes of 28,521 and 8,180 older patients that have heart failure and in hospital in the US and Canada, respectively. Published in November 28, 2005 issue of the Archives of Internal Medicine, it also suggests that 1-year mortality rates are similar for heart failure patients hospitalized in both countries, mortality rates, 32.2% vs. 32.3%. These findings suggest that the U.S and Canadian health systems provide better acute and chronic care, respectively. Could the findings also point to differences in practices, for example, a more intensive approach in the U.S health system including a battery of tests and procedures, compared to a less intensive one in Canada? What are the costs implications of these different approaches as their effects on treatment outcomes are evident in this study specifically that the US patients fared better in the first month but the Canadian patients fared better after the first month? The study also showed that left ventricular ejection fraction evaluations were commoner with U.S than were with Canadian patients during hospitalization, and the former had prescriptions for beta-blockers more frequently than the latter that had prescriptions for angiotensin-converting enzyme inhibitors more frequently than the former. Does this study not tell us something about the ramifications of treatment decisions, and the need for healthcare ICT-backed, evidence-based configuration of optimal healthcare delivery in order to achieve the best short-and long-term clinical outcomes, which would afford us the best chances of reducing healthcare costs? We have illustrated various issues regarding health services delivery and their costs, the roles healthcare ICT could play improving the former, and reducing the latter with heart failure considering it is one of the commonest chronic health conditions that our health systems confront and would even more in the years ahead concerning seniors' health. Besides its important roles in the treatment of this condition and of heart diseases, and all the other chronic health conditions that confront our seniors, these technologies also have a major role to play in preventing these diseases in the first place. They could help prevent them from occurring at all, and if they have, their progression into a worse state and indeed, their sequelae, in short, in the primary, secondary, and tertiary prevention efforts regarding these diseases. Consider the following Heart Outcomes Prevention Evaluation-The Ongoing Outcomes (HOPE-TOO) trial, an extension of the randomized Heart Outcomes Prevention Evaluation (HOPE) trial, published in the March 16, 2005 issue of the Journal of the American Medical Association. The promotion of antioxidants as preventive agents for cancer and cardiovascular disease on the basis that oxidative injury linked to both conditions has been going on for sometime now. Indeed, antioxidants, for example, vitamin E could neutralize free radicals thereby could prevent cell damage and subsequent malignant changes, but findings in studies linking α-tocopherol, its most active form of vitamin E, to prostate, lung, and colon cancer incidence have been at odds, some even showing no benefits at all. α-Tocopherol, the key antioxidant in lipid metabolism, has in animal models lowered blood vessel plaques, and reduced smooth muscle proliferation, and platelet clumping. Indeed, epidemiologic studies have hinted at dietary vitamin E intake reducing the incidence of cardiovascular disease and cancer. However, recent studies (HOPE and HOPE-TOO) the former in which patients observed for 4.5 years did not reveal any protective effect of moderate doses of vitamin E supplementation on cardiovascular outcomes, although it showed a possible protective effect on prostate cancer. HOPE-TOO, an extension of the first study where 174 of the original 267 centers involved in the latter retained 7,030 of the 9,541 patients, did not reveal effect on the incidence of both conditions at 7 years. Indeed, these studies showed that patients in the Vitamin E group in these double-blind, placebo-controlled studies were at higher risk of heart failure, the increased risk, consistent in subgroup analysis by age, sex, history of coronary heart disease, diabetes, and high blood pressure. Considering the promotional efforts mentioned earlier, could many persons, including seniors and baby-boomers currently taking vitamin E in the hope that it could prevent these diseases not know not only that there is no consistent evidence that it does, but that in fact it could put them at risk

137

for heart failure? According to the authors of these studies, "In patients with vascular disease or diabetes mellitus, long-term vitamin E supplementation does not prevent cancer or major cardiovascular events and may increase the risk for heart failure," the authors write. "In conjunction with its lack of efficacy, the potential for harm suggested by our findings strongly supports the view that vitamin E supplements should not be used in patients with vascular disease or diabetes mellitus.... Our findings emphasize the need to thoroughly evaluate all vitamins, other natural products, and complementary medicines in appropriately designed trials before they are widely used for presumed health benefits. " These issues underscore the need for healthcare ICT-backed, targeted health information. There is no doubt about what some would even consider the frenetic pace of the emergence of new medical knowledge, but which no doubt is a good thing. There is in fact already a surfeit of medical information that even the medical professional would likely confess keeping up with is daunting to say the least. Considering the limitations of the memory capabilities of even some of the most profound among us, we could hardly garner blame for our often necessarily deficient health information knowledge base. Further, memory impairment is not an essential accompaniment of, but is no doubt relatively common with age. Hence, we, and in particular our seniors, not only need a regular source of information, but a constant update on this information. Now would it be easier for them to seek this information in say a library or indeed, via the Internet, or receive it in a healthcare ICT-enabled, convenient, contextual, easy-to-assimilate, and targeted format? Besides, even if we expected them to search the Internet for this information could we trust the information they find to be always accurate, current, and unbiased, or might the information slant toward the marketing needs of its provider? Would seniors then be receiving information that would enable them make rational decisions regarding their health or those that might in fact compromise it? What could the ramifications of such flawed decisions also be in terms of their out-of-pocket, healthcare costs for example? Could our seniors and indeed all of us not also benefit from knowing for example that emotional stress could precipitate severe, reversible, left ventricular dysfunction due to an exaggerated sympathetic response as a study published in the February 10, 2005 issue of the New England Journal of Medicine showed[13]. As Ilan S. Wittstein, MD, from Johns Hopkins University in Baltimore, Maryland, noted, "The potentially lethal consequences of emotional stress are deeply rooted in folk wisdom, as reflected by phrases such as 'scared to death' and 'a broken heart'". He added, "In the past decade, cardiac contractile abnormalities and heart failure have been reported after acute emotional stress, but the mechanism remains unknown". The authors employed coronary angiography and serial echocardiography, to evaluate 19 patients that presented with left ventricular dysfunction after sudden emotional stress, five of who had endomyocardial biopsy, and another five, cardiac magnetic resonance imaging to identify myocardial necrosis. The researchers assessed all participants with electrocardiography, did cardiac enzymes, echocardiography, and coronary angiography. Termed myocardial stunning, severe emotional stress causes cardiac contractile abnormalities and heart failure for a variety of reasons such as epicardial coronary artery spasm as seen in persons with increased sympathetic tone due to mental stress; microvascular spasm within the heart consequent upon a sudden release of stress hormones; and direct injury to cardiac myocytes. Could the findings of this study not help some individuals to control their emotions more effectively, and reduce the risk of heart failure? Could information on the role of obesity as an independent risk factor for the development of heart failure not help increase awareness of the need to combat obesity? Would this not also help reduce the prevalence of obesity-related diseases, which have reached epidemic levels in many countries including the U.S[14]? The strong link between obesity and the increased risk of developing cardiovascular (CV) diseases such as atherosclerosis, hypertension, and stroke is not in doubt. There is also research evidence to support the wide variety of heart diseases linked to obesity, such as left ventricular (LV) hypertrophy, even cardiomyopathy[15]. Could knowledge of this information not also help increase awareness of the dangers of overweight and obesity, and would intensifying efforts to deliver this information to those that need them not help reduce the prevalence of these conditions and overall help reduce healthcare costs? The numbers of new research with valuable health information is legion some of this information capable of changing certain practices some people engage in that are detrimental to their health, early enough to make a significant difference to even whether they survive or they do not. In other words, we must find ways to get the information out to the public as soon as practicable, the question being which other means could enable us do that most cost-effectively and efficiently than healthcare ICT. It is difficult to overemphasize the need for targeted health information, because it is perhaps the most efficient way by which we could achieve our dual goals of qualitative healthcare delivery, cost-effectively, regardless of the funding model of the health system. It is even the more crucial for us to appreciate this fact considering our increasing consumer-centric health systems. How could we say that the consumer that lacks information on making rational decisions about his/her health is a discerning one? Could such lack of information not in fact lead the consumer to make flawed choices that might compromises his/her health and increase healthcare costs? As our discussion so far has shown, our efforts to control healthcare costs simultaneously delivering qualitative healthcare have to be multifaceted in approach, involving the examination of a variety of issues but also for example, of the individual as a payer in a general consideration of payer issues. We also need to examine healthcare provider issues, including remuneration, and incentives, for example to purchase healthcare ICT, which would enable the full exploitation of the technologies offerings, progress in medical and technological knowledge, and systems and policies issues, among others. We need to understand the theoretical underpinnings of these various issues, in order to appreciate our real life observations, and to be able to take the necessary steps to channel these observations toward achieving our healthcare delivery and cost containment goals.

Healthcare costs drivers would qualify as generic and specific, the former that

would apply to all health systems and the latter those peculiar to a health system based on local characteristics such as disease prevalence patterns, demographics, even diet. For example, total hip and total knee replacement today are less costly than they were a quarter century ago, for example, although the costs of implants are on the rise, which applies in general to the markets for these products. On the other hand, the factors involved in the reasons for the questioning of the value of public defibrillators are likely to have a local flavor. A Canadian study presented on May 19, 2006 at the annual meeting of the Society for Academic Emergency Medicine, in San Francisco, has questioned the increasing public access to automated external heart defibrillators, which the researchers to be cost-effective only in three types of locations, namely casinos, non-acute hospitals and nursing homes. Dr. Valerie J. De Maio one of the researchers noted, "Less than 15 percent of cardiac arrests occur in public venues. PAD (public access defibrillation) programs that target public venues are unlikely to lead to significant overall survival benefit." The researchers studied almost 7,700 cardiac arrest incidents from 1995 to 2000, including the costs and life expectancy of treating patients with versus without on-site defibrillator by location. Using a threshold of $50,000 per annum of life gained, they found that the locations that met the cost-effectiveness criteria were only casinos ($542), non-acute hospitals ($30,750), and nursing homes ($45,926), while costs in others, for example, shopping malls ($67,690), hotels ($143,530), restaurants and bars ($347,954), medical offices ($955,614), and stadiums and fairgrounds ($1,910,193), did not. We need to examine these figures, and find out the possible reasons for the variations, in order to review and probably change the relevant policies, hence future investments in these defibrillators and to determine where to locate them. Perhaps, we might even want to examine other options. For example, Dr Maio recommended that rather than locate defibrillators at large public centers, "there is a much greater opportunity to improve survivability by focusing on the delivery of good-quality basic CPR and programs designed to increase awareness among the community," which underscores the point regarding the need for healthcare ICT diffusion. The more widespread use of healthcare ICT among healthcare stakeholders would no doubt facilitate targeted health information dissemination including innovative program development to achieve the sort of health education goals that Dr. Maio recommended, among others. Regardless of whether it is generic or specific, we need to analyze and understand why healthcare costs are increasing relentlessly, in order to find the right solutions to them. The average total hip or total knee procedure, for example, used to be up to two and a half hours, the patient in hospital for over two weeks, versus now that the procedure takes three quarters of an hour and the patient in hospital overnight or perhaps a day or two more. What does this higher OR turnover time, number of procedures per day per OR, and much shorter hospital stays mean in terms of overall costs? Combined with improved rehabilitation efforts, could prognosis even long-term be sufficiently favorable to discountenance the increasing costs of implants? Here again, we are looking at the overall cost structure when considering healthcare costs in order to see which of the variables involved is in fact the culprit in an observed high cost situation for example, and in fact to determine whether the overall benefits of the cost driver would outweigh the costs in the end. Such an analysis would involve not just a global look at these variables but also their contributions to costs in the short and long-terms. This issue is particularly germane to our discussion on the need for more widespread healthcare ICT diffusion in our health systems, and at all healthcare stakeholder levels. It also underscores the point we made about the irrelevance of the funding of the health system to our realizing the full benefits of implementing these technologies on such a large scale in the health system in achieving the dual objectives mentioned above. In fact, we also hold that as with the underlying principle of free market operations inform us, that everyone will be a winner in the end. Consider for example a situation where medical and technological knowledge makes us understand the underlying pathologies of diseases better, the family doctor has access to new treatment modalities quicker and patients' health information when needed being hooked up with the Internet and regional electronic health records systems, he/she is thus able to treat the patient more effectively. The patient has access to valuable health information that assists him/her in maintaining improvement, and no longer requires frequent hospitalizations, as before, and needs fewer and less expensive medications and lab investigations. The family doctor gains a reputation for excellence, more patients enroll in the practice, and income increases. The hospital has fewer wait lists, reconfigures its value proposition, and makes revenues from delivering new services or strengthening those that its clients need, and the pharmaceutical companies, which are still selling drugs, do the same in a continual market analysis and product and market diversification that every business organization must perform from time to time. Therefore, no one loses, in the end. Indeed, the corollary of the business dictum referred to above is that there would be no exchange were this not the expectation of the parties involved. In other words, in a true market situation, everyone expects to gain something, and ideally, on the aggregate, this is the case. By developing our ambulatory/community/ domiciliary services backed by healthcare ICT, we might be able to manage many individuals with chronic medical conditions in these different settings than in a hospital thereby saving costs, but this would require investing in a variety of healthcare ICT upfront in order to monitor and manage these chronic illnesses successfully. This is because one of the chief requirements of an effective multidisciplinary team is communication, and information sharing. Even in hospitals, the need for such activities and processes is immense not to mention in multiple settings outside the hospital. These technologies for example telemedicine could facilitate the examination of and recommendations on appropriate treatment options for a number of conditions that seniors have including arthritis, and diabetes, which obviates the need for hospital visits and stays and their associated costs. These changes in orientation of health services delivery would most certainly affect the future of hospitals, as we currently know them. To be sure, hospitals are not all going to disappear overnight, alt hough some of them that cannot justify their continued existence, in business terms, would eventually be moribund and extinct. To prevent this fate, we are going to see more of the current cost-saving strategies hospitals are employing such as competitive bidding, capitation, rationalizing vendor base, gain sharing, seeking discount prices, mergers, and super-specialization, among others. Hospitals would have to collaborate with their suppliers in reducing costs, and examine ways to improve volume, while not sacrificing quality, or compromising outcomes. Indeed, health authorities could participate in promoting quality in a number of different ways, for example, the Swedes have a national joint registry, which tracks success rates on orthopedic devices, information that could inform investment in one or another such device, with perhaps significant costs implications.

There is no disputing the important roles of healthcare in any society, but none

either regarding the need for the health system to be viable in order to meet these roles. Consider for example what would happen to healthcare delivery to seniors were Medicare to constitute the projected 9.2% of the gross domestic product (GDP) of the U.S in 2050, half attributed to an increasingly aging population, the other half, healthcare costs increases above GDP growth rates. Given this scenario, at current general revenue financing levels, there will only be up to 3.8% of the GDP available for public health spending, which means slashing health services by more than in half by 2050 in order to match health spending with revenue forecasts. What would this mean for the health of our seniors and do we want it to happen? Certainly not, and which is why we need to discuss the issues pertaining to healthcare costs and find ways to achieve our dual objectives mentioned earlier. In the U.S for example, we should be seeking ways to reduce health spending by almost 50% by 2050. How could we do this? One way is if seniors had fewer illnesses for which to require treatment. In other words, the fewer the number of comorbidities, the less the expenditures on the senior, and indeed, some experts contend that lifetime medical spending for the average person would fall by 17% [16]. Does this not mean we should make an effort to reduce comorbidities, for example reducing the prevalence of overweight and obesity, smoking, and alcohol dependence among seniors? Could healthcare ICT not help in facilitating programs that could enable us achieve this goal? Should we not continue to develop even more sophisticated healthcare ICT that would enable seniors to monitor their blood pressure and sugar at home, which could result in prevention of high blood pressure and diabetes, or in better controlling them? Should we not invest in information and communications technologies that would make our public health systems work better, with resulting better disease surveillance and higher chances of our health promotion and disease prevention effort succeeding? On the other hand, we must recognize that there are some age-related diseases. These diseases, which one could say are simply due to the " wear and tear " on our systems with time, and until researchers find the answers to cellular regeneration, as they could with the progress so far made in many areas including in our nervous system, we have to live with, will remain healthcare cost drivers. These diseases, for example arthritis, coupled with limitations in activities of daily living (ADLs) or instrumental activities of daily living (IADLs), both on which seniors spend twice as much as those without limitation, constitute significant portions of the almost $90,000 some experts estimated even the healthy 65-year old would spend on healthcare over the rest of his/her life. We must also recognize that death, and the illnesses that precede it are costly, that these end-of-life issues cost as much as a 25% of lifetime medical costs for seniors incurred in their last year of existence, and almost 30% of annual Medicare spending incurred on persons that will expire in a year. Indeed, the older an individual lives, the less these costs, twice less for example, for one that died at over 90 years than another who did before seventy, because the former often succumbs to less costly illnesses such as pneumonia, than the younger seniors do. This means that the longer we keep our seniors alive, the less en-of-life costs we incur. End-of-life costs are thus also legitimate costs issues that we must focus on in our efforts to reduce healthcare costs. In addition, should we therefore not do whatever we could to keep our seniors living longer? Indeed, this is the natural order of things that we only need to promote by eschewing risk factors for ill health, a message that healthcare ICT could play a pivotal role in helping us disseminate successfully. As we noted earlier in our discussion, there are issues relating to information asymmetry, with seniors in particular lacking crucial health information that we need to recognize and address. We want to ask on what health issues and services are both healthy and unhealthy seniors are spending money for example, and could information asymmetry be at play here with seniors in both categories either misinformed or inadequately informed about what is good for their health, and the choices they make regarding treatment providers, and the treatment the seniors receive? Would these problems not have adverse implications for example on the overall health of both groups, with even the healthy seniors spilling over into the unhealthy group, which latter stand the risk of their health deteriorating further? Would these developments not worsen the health status of seniors overall and increase healthcare costs and health spending across board? Would exploring these issues not indicate the need for more energetic approaches to rectifying this information asymmetry, which healthcare ICT could assist in achieving cost-effectively? Regarding the illnesses that are in essence inevitable with old age, and which we must deal with, could we not do so more cost-effectively? Could we not substitute angioplasty for more costly bypass surgery, for example? Could not use less expensive but just as effective generic medications instead of brand names? Could we not use effective, healthcare ICT-backed, evidence-based treatments thus reducing hospitalization rates, and even the frequency of physician visits? Some would argue that some of these suggestions might reduce unit costs only to lead to increase volume, hence more overall costs. However, the question is if those that constitute the extra volume previously had the medical problem for which they received treatment, and if so, why they only came up for treatment or received treatment with the introduction of these suggested measures. Is there something wrong with treatment substitution? The question really should be if, following the introduction of a new inexpensive, day-procedure, everyone should have appendectomy, or prostatectomy, simply because these organs are redundant and could eventually spell health trouble. This does not mean that we should overlook the long-term effect of treatment expansion, though, as the reduction in the pool of the untreated would lead in the end to fewer persons to which to expand treatment. This scenario might work well in a publicly funded health system such as in Canada where some might have concerns about the " moral hazard" issue raised by the question regarding the "problem" with treatment substitution. It also underscores our point in this discussion that investing in innovative healthcare ICT in such systems, even with no obvious immediate pecuniary advantages is in fact still economically viable, even if more so in the long term. In a privately funded health system such as in the U.S, the mechanisms are quite different for how we are in fact going to end up with the same result, that is, achieving our dual objectives of providing qualitative healthcare cost-effectively, although the fundamental underpinning of these different mechanisms, the widespread implementation and use of healthcare ICT, remains the same. There are going to be innovative ideas on healthcare delivery that would have far-reaching effects on our ability to achieve the dual goals mentioned earlier in the near future. In Canada, for example, there are those that advocate the establishment of a parallel private health system, which if it did eventually happen would change the dynamics of the players in the country's health system significantly, but which irrespective of these changes would reflect the key role of process improvement in making any health system work. Even without a parallel private health system in place, the country's health system would benefit immensely from widespread healthcare ICT implementation, which the country's health authorities clearly recognize, as its investments in a number of health-related ICT projects worth about $1.5 billion between 1997 and 2003, indicates. Physical inactivity alone costs the Canadian health care system roughly $2.1 billion yearly in direct health care costs, the estimated yearly economic burden, $5.3 billion. The country spent $126 million on healthcare ICT via Canada Health Infoway in 2004, and planned to spend $195 million more in 2005. Canadian provinces are also investing significantly in healthcare ICT. Alberta earmarked $2.6 million from its Telehealth Clinical Services Grant Fund to twenty-one new telehealth programs in 2005. It also has a $66 million Alberta Physician Office System Program, in association with the Alberta Medical Association, and under which, every doctor in the province could receive $7,700 in each of four years to install, train in, and begin to use electronic medical records (EMR) in his/her practice. Over 50% of its doctors have responded positively to this initiative. Such incentive programs should constitute an integral part of our efforts to promote the widespread diffusion and use of healthcare ICT, if we were ever to derive the desired benefits from these technologies that could move us forward toward achieving the dual objectives. Ontario is investing $57 million over a five-year period to support patient care using healthcare ICT. The province also plans to invest another $45 million on added diagnostic equipments, including mobile devices, between 2003 and 2006. All other Canadian provinces and territories are committed to implementing healthcare ICT to facilitate healthcare delivery. With the estimated annual economic burden of illness, disability, and death due to chronic diseases in Canada over $80 billion, the costs of unhealthy eating alone in the country in 2000, $6.3 billion, including direct health care costs of $1.8 billion, and its overall health spending increasing, do these ICT investments not make perfect sense? Many other developed countries such as the U.K, Australia, New Zealand, France, are also investing in these technologies significantly. According to the World Health Organization (WHO), it is possible to prevent or delay over 90% of type 2 diabetes and 80% of coronary heart disease, with proper nutrition, regular physical activity, quitting cigarette smoking, and effective stress management. Could healthcare ICT-backed preventive initiatives not help in this regard? Some might argue that people already know about the health dangers of unhealthy lifestyles, which though true does not preclude delivering the messages to them in different ways, using innovative technologies, and emphasizing different aspects of such health promotion programs that are relevant to the particular population receiving the messages. The point here is that health promotion and disease prevention efforts should be "work-in-progress," and one we could never give up on in view of new research findings emerging from time to time for example on changing disease patterns and natural histories, and of the effectiveness or otherwise of our ongoing efforts. Even if our previous efforts had succeeded to a certain extent, should we not update them to improve their effectiveness? Recent research findings in Quebec for example showed that showing pictures of the pathological effects of cigarette smoking on the teeth and lungs on cigarette packs did not discourage chronic smokers from quitting the habit, but did to a certain extent, individuals that have not started the habit. In the first place, is discouraging young people, who are most prone to picking up the habit from doing so not an achievement? Secondly, should the results of this research not prompt us to ask further questions and perhaps initiate additional research to find answers to them regarding why the campaign failed to discourage chronic smokers? Do some of these smokers for example believe that smoking would help them eat less, hence lose weight, and keep their weights down? Do some view smoking as some kind of reward after an effort at a task? Do some of them use smoking to relief anxiety in relationships under strain? Is smoking for many serving a multiplicity of purposes? Are there biological factors involved in smoking? These and many other questions need answers in order to help these chronic smokers quit the habit before it is too late. This is why our health promotion and disease prevention campaigns must be ongoing and regularly modified to incorporate new research findings. Is it likely that contextualizing such messages would make a difference in their acceptance, for example emphasizing the turn-off of "yellow, nicotine-stained teeth", and "cigarette breath" to young people contemplating their first kiss? Should we not be delivering targeted and contextualized health information on cigarettes to chronic smokers debunking the myths about cigarettes that fuel their habits with hard, scientific facts? Should we not be doing the same for those dependent on other substances, for example alcohol, cocaine, crystal meth, and others? Would healthcare ICT not help substantially in effecting these initiatives? Do the examples not speak to the benefits of targeted health information dissemination?

As noted earlier, our efforts to reduce healthcare costs must be multidimensional,

and innovative. In the U.S for example, one such innovative approach to healthcare delivery is retail medical care, and it is gaining increasing currency quite rapidly, embraced by the healthcare consumer and entrepreneur alike. At Wal-Mart, CVS, and a host of other chain stores, walk-in health clinics are emerging to counter the expense and hassle of full-service doctors' offices and the pricey and frosty last resort of the ER. With patients paying just $30 for a flu shot, $45 for the treatment of an ear infection or other routine services, their price lists posted for all to see, should it be surprising that health consumers are queuing to visit nurse practitioners in independently operated clinics in these stores, which also have in-store pharmacies to fill the prescriptions? The U.S now has about a hundred of these clinics spread across the country, with many more on the way, established by entrepreneurs from disparate backgrounds that range from the health to the hospitality industry, the concept of "consumer-driven healthcare", the underlying principle behind their efforts. Essentially this model implies higher out-of-pocket medical costs with mass-market prospects, with even some health insurers embracing its cost saving potential, not to mention those uninsured for whom, these clinics are in general more affordable than most other options, such as the for-profit storefront clinics that offered a full range of physician-provided medical services to walk-in consumers. These newer clinics also offer an opportunity to receive the healthcare that they otherwise lack, and many, including doctors, believe that these clinics are here to stay, for one because they are likely to be under pressure from the store chains, who have put their name on the line, to deliver qualitative services as well. With the potential to change profoundly the approach to primary care in the U.S., retail clinics are the effects of changes in employer-sponsored insurance benefits discussed earlier, with people having to fund more or all of their own health costs, and public displeasure at the increasing costs, and some would say inefficiency of traditional health services. Licensed nurse practitioners run most of the clinics, and most have advanced training and referral arrangements with local doctors for cases that are beyond their expertise, here again, communication with who might be urgent and life saving, hence the need for even these retail clinics to hook up with the regional health information network (RHIN), to facilitate information flow. The usual presence of a pharmacy store within the complex makes filling prescriptions much easier although some doctors contend that the clinic-pharmacy link could create conflicts of interest, and work against the patient's interests. There is no doubt about the possibilities of some abuse, which is why these retail clinics need some oversight. This could expose and prevent such abuses, allowing patients to continue to benefit from the services that these clinics provide, which no doubt complement the others in the overall health system, and improve accessibility to care, a major condition for us to achieve the dual objectives mentioned earlier. Indeed, with more of these clinics operational, market forces would further result in lower pricing, hence make them even more affordable and accessible, while and with regular supervision, they are also delivering qualitative services within their competencies. There is no doubt that retail clinics fill a need, in particular providing acute health care to people mildly ill persons whose only option at the time might be an ER. Because they have a limited scope, no requirement for costly medical equipment or office space, retail clinics have lower startup and maintenance costs than many doctors offices, particularly with the nurse practitioner paid between $30 and $45, versus the doctor s $65 or much more an hour, hence we should expect many more to open. They are also apparently profitable for their owners. Retail clinics are in fact starting to take different forms, some, with more sophisticated service offerings than others do. Solantic clinics, for example, have doctors on staff and offer a variety of services including X-rays at $90 each, and their prices are higher for routine services than the other retail clinics. The direction and the full impact of these clinics on the U.S health services will unfold no doubt in the months and years ahead. That retail clinics work in the U.S does not mean that it would in other countries particularly those such as in Canada with a different health funding system. Nonetheless, each health system needs to innovate with regard health services delivery, developing delivery models that could help achieve the dual objectives we mentioned earlier. These innovative practices could be at any level of the healthcare delivery chain, namely, primary, secondary, and tertiary. Retail clinics are examples of innovative healthcare delivery models, the concept of "complementarity", and regionalization, mentioned earlier, examples at the secondary/tertiary levels. We could also conceptualize these innovations in public health terms, namely, primary, secondary, and tertiary, prevention initiatives, some of which we have also mentioned. There could also be a mix of services and public health approaches, with retail clinics for example offering health promotion and disease prevention services, for examples, gyms and wellness centers perhaps even targeted at specific populations, for examples, seniors, females, even youngsters, which even service outlets at the secondary and tertiary levels, could offer. Underlying these various considerations and approaches must be the efficient and effective delivery of qualitative and affordable services, which is where healthcare ICT becomes crucial as a facilitator. To be sure, with the increasing emphasis on population health, which itself is tacit recognition of what the overall goal of healthcare delivery ought to be, we should increase our efforts in improving public health services, considering that we could manipulate many of the factors that determine health or ill health via appropriate public health measures. In fact, healthcare systems worldwide confront increasing pressure to develop health policy and program initiatives that reallocate more institutional resources to public health programs of different foci, but all essentially aimed at improving the health of all. It is indubitable that healthcare ICT reduces the transaction costs of and is the pivot of the success of many of these public health initiatives. Our efforts to contain healthcare costs must also consider developments in healthcare beyond our borders. There is little doubt that with the developments in the airline industry such as the new Airbus A380, with the capacity to transport over 500 persons across the globe in one trip, it is, simply put becoming easier for us to carry diseases along with us back and forth on our business trips or vacations. Playing our part in world health affairs, for example, participating in and completing international agreements on global efforts to combat diseases, for example, Avian flu, is an investment in our own health as well, albeit, indirectly. Even if the diseases we help to control are not contagious, we are, by our generosity, assisting our fellow beings in being healthy, hence productive in their societies, and be able to participate effectively in world trade and economic exchanges. This no doubt would create a more fertile milieu for international trade by increasing the numbers of buyers and sellers, and of course the goods and services to exchange, from all of which our economies would benefit ultimately. By benefiting from such buoyant world economic climate, we would not only be able to develop our economies, but they would become more sustainable, and we would be able to offer our citizens even better healthcare. This way, our citizens become healthier and even more productive, and more competitive on the world economic stage. With economic prosperity in many countries of the world, there would be less internal agitation and more peace and stability in countries, and in the world at large. Competition on the economic stage would keep us busy enough to meet our instinctive need for action, and as the above discussion shows, with everyone guaranteed a piece. We have sufficient reasons to invest in healthcare ICT as the above discussion also shows. These technologies are the chief "de-drivers" of costs in our quest to achieve our dual healthcare delivery objectives. They also as we have seen constitute the fundamental enablers of societal progress, peace, and harmony. By freeing up valuable resources we could invest in education, we build a legion of intellectuals who would upgrade our technology base and make us even more competitive. To underscore the need for an international perspective on health the European Commission recently called for Proposals 2006 Programme of Community Action in the field of Public Health (2003-2008) to implement the priority actions defined in the Work Plan 2006 of the Public H ealth programme (2003-2008). The 6 May 2000 presented the first European Health strategy and proposed the Public Health programme. The May 2000 communication, with support from the public health programme, resulted in the development of public health activities and to improving links to other health-related policies. Since then, there had been the establishment of a European Centre for Disease Prevention and Control (ECDC), cross-border co-operation between health systems, and health determinants, tackled, and "The Community's health information system provides a key mechanism underpinning the development of health policy." [17] The EU Health Forum offers organizations active in health the opportunity to express their views on health policy to the EU, whose health policy emphasizes inter-state collaboration in particular on cross-border issues for example, patient mobility. The Commission launched a review process of the May 2000 Health Strategy in 2004, to examine how well it meeting its goals and would, the new broader objective of "enabling good health for all". As the Commission noted, healthcare ICT plays a crucial role in implementing public health initiatives, and additionally, in their success. One important aspect of the ability of these technologies to deliver in this context is for the governments of these various collaborating countries to agree on the technicalities of information transfer. People are becoming ever-more mobile, and in countries with reciprocal trade and other agreements, this need to harmonize technology standards as noted earlier, becomes quite urgent. Thus, for example, someone who is on vacation in Brussels from Paris could access healthcare in the former readily, with the treating physicians also able to access his/her health information at the point of care (POC), and in real time. Such ready access could save many lives and of course healthcare costs. However, without the widespread implementation of healthcare ICT in either country, such possibly life-saving, ready access to health information might not materialize. Furthermore, even with the offices of the patient's doctors in Paris and Brussels automated, they might still be unable to exchange the patient's health information because the technologies in both countries are not interoperable, for example, because the countries have not agreed on interoperability standards. With software and other healthcare ICT developing their products using disparate specifications, and standards that often only apply locally, we could never achieve the sort of collaboration that the European Commission seeks, even among its member states. This lack of internationally viable standards will likely compromise healthcare delivery within countries too, as for example, the health of the patient, whose stroke say that he/she had in Brussels, has worsened because of delay in the doctors in Paris obtaining his/her health records, is much worse back, for the same reason. Only this time, the delay in accessing information, reversed. This state of affairs would not only have adversely affected the health of this person, who might be a senior trying to enjoy retirement visiting a few places, creating misery and agony for him/her and the family, but perhaps also created a chronic debilitating state with significant cost implications for long-term care. It is likely that these problems are not as far-fetched as they might sound at first, and that they constitute significant cost drivers for our health systems, and need rectifying. Thus, addressing these and other technology issues such as product certification, to ensure uniformity of quality, for example, is also a critical aspect of our cost containment measures. Many of the processes that these technologies facilitate are " mission critical " in the health field, and the last thing we want is to have these technologies being cost drivers rather than "de-drivers," which if by failure in the middle of an operation or procedure, or delaying the receipt of some vital drug allergy information, morbidities and mortalities rise, they become. Furthermore, it is important for the healthcare providers that we are trying to convince to purchase and implement these technologies to know that their total cost of ownership (TCO) would not literally be flying through the roof, due to lingering maintenance costs. Indeed, hospital administrators these days have to choose from an increasing variety of healthcare ICT and major medical equipments, posing tough challenges for customary capital allocation processes, which certification could help ease. This becomes even more important considering the increasing roles of the rules the Centers for Medicare and Medicaid Services (CMS) in the U.S, for example, and similar bodies and private insurers elsewhere, set on coverage and reimbursement. Yet, healthcare ICT and medical equipment acquisition is an exercise healthcare providers must engage in, in the present dispensation of healthcare delivery. Certification also means that we would have involved vendors in our efforts to achieve the dual objectives if they played their parts in ensuring they develop high quality products, as the relationship of such products to high quality healthcare delivery is no doubt direct. There are other non-technical issues than we have discussed, for example that of the remuneration of healthcare providers that also drive healthcare costs. This issue is quite complex and warrants in-depth exploration, not only because it is a major cost driver, but also because it is at the core of the success of our efforts. Imagine for example that all doctors refused to work because of poor remuneration as they did in Germany for two weeks recently. Indeed, German doctors have reportedly been leaving the country en masse to seek "greener pastures" abroad and to escape the crippling bureaucracy in the country, an estimated 2,700, 2,600, 700, and 650 in the U.S, Britain, Sweden, and Norway, respectively. Many German doctors also do weekend locum tenens in Britain and other countries to supplement their incomes. The annual salaries of hospital doctors in $U.S adjusted for purchasing power, are 267,993; 203132; 175,155; 127,285; 116077; 81,414; 73,236; and 67,785 in the U.S, Australia, Netherlands, Britain, France, Italy, Denmark, and Spain, respectively, compared to 56,455, in Germany[18]. With just about 50% of medical student ending up practicing doctors in Germany, many rather as bureaucrats in the health service, working in industry, or emigrating, the adverse effects of these developments on the country's health system are unquestionable. Even when doctors plus their standard salary receive extra payments for shift work, medical reports, and a percentage of the money from the treatment of private payments, they still earn much less than their counterparts in many developed countries, despite that they likely work longer hours, and that the country spends €240 billion spent on health services. There is also the issue of the often-overbearing head doctors and hospital administrators, and that of sharing of private treatment payments. The medical law in the western state of Hesse, for example, mandates head physicians to share out about 80% of proceeds from private patients to the clinic and to the doctors involved in treating the patient. However, some head physicians do not share the money out this way, resulting in sometime-serious rancor that contributes to the reasons some doctors leave the country, related to which is many rural doctors not able to find successors to hand their surgeries to when they retire. According to experts, the country is likely going to waste more than €1 billion of university costs training medical students only 7,000 out of 12,000 of which complete their training, and many of those that did emigrating. These developments thus also have implications for the country's wider economy and indeed, for those of the host countries for their émigré doctors, who face increasing competition from the newcomers. This example illustrates the complexity of the issue of doctors' remuneration and their ramifications, hence the need to address them cautiously, objectively and in detail. Indeed, it also needs dealing with in the context of a country's health system, and other factors. In other words, whether a country chooses capitation, fee-for-service, pay-per-performance or any remuneration principle should be well thought-out, and predicated on a variety of local factors and developments in the global health arena. An aspect of this issue is that regarding incentives for healthcare providers to purchase and implement healthcare ICT, as Alberta province does as noted earlier. Whether we are talking about Medicare, or Medicaid, in the U.S., Medicare, in Canada, or the NHS, in the U.K., the widespread implementation of healthcare ICT is sine qua non for realizing the promise of these technologies for the overall health system. The issues relating to healthcare costs are legion, and vary from country to country, but the main issue concerning the relationship between healthcare ICT and costs apply to all countries, and it is that these technologies could play a vital role in helping us achieve the dual objectives of delivering qualitative healthcare to all, cost-effectively. Common to all countries and health systems is also that the realization of these objectives depends on the widespread diffusion and utilization of these technologies. The real task then is for each country to establish the mechanisms for the diffusion of the healthcare ICT most suited to its specific needs and milieu and for healthcare providers and other healthcare stakeholders to determine for which processes in the healthcare delivery chain they need to implement the technologies. With the required healthcare ICT deployed ubiquitously, the health system is set to deliver on its promise of actualizing the dual objectives of qualitative healthcare delivery to all, simultaneously reducing healthcare costs.

References

1. Goldman DP. et al., "Consequences of Health Trends and Medical Innovation for the Elderly of the Future," *Health Affairs,* 26 September 2005, content.healthaffairs.org/cgi/content/abstract/hlthaff.w5.r5; and J. Bhattacharya et al., "Technological Advances in Cancer and Future Spending by the Sderly," *Health Affairs,* 26 September 2005, content.healthaffairs.org/cgi/content/abstract/hlthaff.w5.r53.

2. Smith, C., Cowan, C., Heftier, S., National Health Spending in 2004: Recent Slowdown Led By Prescription Drug Spending *Health Affairs* 25, no. 1 (2006): 186-196]

3. Romano M. Pros and cons of certificates: American Health Planning Association directory suggests that certificate-of-need process is regulatory in theory, not in practice. *Mod Healthc.* 2003; 33:4‾5

4. Popescu I, Vaughan-Sarrazin MS, Rosenthal GE. Certificate of need regulations and use of coronary revascularization after acute myocardial infarction. *JAMA.* 2006; 295:2141-2147.

5. Krumholz HM, Anderson JL, Brooks NH, et al, American College of Cardiology/ American Heart Association Task Force on Performance Measures. ACC/AHA clinical performance measures for adults with ST-elevation and non-ST- elevation myocardial infarction: a report of the American College of Cardiology/American Heart Association Task Force on Performance Measures. *J Am Coll Cardiol.* 2006; 47:236 265.

6. Antman EM, Anbe DT, Armstrong PW, et al, American College of Cardiology; American Heart Association; Canadian Cardiovascular Society. ACC/AHA guidelines for the management of patients with ST-elevation myocardial infarction: executive summary: a report of the American College of Cardiology/American Heart Association Task Force on Practice Guidelines. *J Am Coll Cardiol.* 2004; 44:671⁻719.

7. Hannan EL, Wu C, Walford G, et al. Volume-outcome relationships for percutaneous coronary interventions in the stent era. *Circulation.* 2005; 112:1171⁻1179.

8. Available at: http://www.americanheart.org Accessed May 20, 2006

9. Moss AJ, Zareba W, Hall WJ, et al. Prophylactic implantation of a defibrillator in patients with myocardial infarction and reduced ejection fraction. *N Engl J Med.* 2002; 346(12):877–883.

10. St. John Sutton MG, Plappert T, Abraham WT, et al. Effect of cardiac resynchronization therapy on left ventricular size and function in chronic heart failure. *Circulation.* 2003; 107:1985⁻1990.

11. Seow H, Phillips CO, Rich MW, et al. Isolation of health services research from practice and policy: the example of chronic heart failure management. *J Am Geriatr Soc* 2006 Mar; 54(3):535-540.

12. *Arch Intern Med* 2005; 165:2486-2492.

13. *N Engl J Med.* 2005; 352:539-548

14. Must A, Spadano J, Coakley EH, et al. The disease burden associated with overweight and obesity. *JAMA.* 1999; 282: 1523⁻1529.

15. Messerli FH. Cardiopathy of obesity—a not-so-Victorian disease. *N Engl J Med.* 1986; 314: 378–380.

16. Joyce GF. et al., "The Lifetime Burden of Chronic Disease among the Elderly,"
Health *Affairs,* 26 September 2005,
content.healthaffairs.org/cgi/content/abstract/hlthaff.w5.rl8.

17. Available at:

http://ec.europa.eu/comm/health/ph_overview/strategy/health_strategy_en.htm
Accessed on May 21, 2006

18. National Economic Research Associates Economic Consultants. Available at:
http://service.spiegel.de/cache/international/0,1518,399537,00.html
Accessed on May 21, 2006

ICT and the Disease Prevention Paradigm

A new World Bank report titled, *Health Financing Revisited-A Practitioners Guide*,

raises major concerns about the financial quagmire in which healthcare systems worldwide are due to soaring healthcare costs, simultaneously struggling to deal with the HIV/AIDS crisis and avert the chances of human bird flu pandemic. The report, released on May 25, 2006, also questioned the prospects of current global efforts to achieve core Millennium Development Goals including expanding the reach of healthcare systems to improve the health of millions of the world's poorest people by 2015. The report noted the huge mismatch between countries' health financial needs and their current health spending, essentially painting a dismal picture of the healthcare system, nationally and worldwide. According to the report, global health spending was $3.2 trillion, about 10% of global gross domestic product in 2002, just 12% of which went to low- and middle-income countries. The report also noted that problems with health systems in countries, eventually constrain productivity and economic growth. The report observed that high-income countries spend about 100 times more on health per person than low-income countries, over 50% of funds the latter expends from out-of-pocket payments by the healthcare consumer, a recipe for financial ruin for people that struggle with subsistence, a situation demographic changes might in fact worsen over time. It is uncertain if the projected growth in world population from 6 billion to 7.5 billion by 2020, most of this growth expected in developing countries, the population in 50 of the world's poorest nations billed to double by 2050 would be a "demographic gift" of speedier economic growth or a "demographic curse" of greater unemployment and social turmoil. The World Bank official that made this observation added that this would eventually depend on government policies that promote economic and labor force growth. In this regard, the report made some key revelations regarding the direction of global and national health expenditures, noting that demographic changes alone will increase healthcare spending by 2 to 3% annually in most low- and middle-income countries over the next 20 years. It also noted that regionally, this would increase health-care spending needs by 50% in Latin America and the Caribbean, 45% in South Asia, and 14% in Europe and Central Asia, the highest rise, 62%, in the Middle East and North Africa. With regard the Millennium Development Goals for health, the report noted that despite that health aid increased to over $10 billion in 2003 from $2.6 billion in 1990, current estimates show the requirement of between three and seven times that much to achieve the goals. With three million people killed by HIV/AIDS in 2005 alone in poor countries, despite a significant increase in aid for health, and these countries still struggling to avoid a human bird-flu pandemic, their situation is clearly dire. The report acknowledged that funding from private foundations was almost 20% of total health aid, and advocated the increase in development aid by the international community. It specifically noted that "Many donor efforts have increased transaction costs, and fragmented health service delivery", which clearly indicates the need for process improvement that the deployment of appropriate healthcare ICT could rectify. The report acknowledged, "there is no single road" for countries intent on providing good health-care services at the lowest cost, with a variety of options available such as national health service systems, social health insurance funds, private voluntary health insurance, community-based health insurance, or direct purchases by consumers. Nonetheless, there is no doubt that such appropriate implementation and utilization of healthcare ICT could help achieve these dual goals even in these poor countries. However, they would need to tailor the technologies so deployed to their needs and within the context of their institutional, technical, and other relevant infrastructures. They would also need to confront the challenges of reforming their health financing systems to create enough operating budgets, and assure access to qualitative and effective healthcare by their peoples while protecting them against poverty, compounded by high out-of-pocket healthcare costs, goals they could also achieve exploiting the immense opportunities that healthcare ICT offers. Besides the U.S., according to the report, almost all high-income countries have achieved universal or near universal health coverage, which developing countries could use as models. There are certainly no quick fixes to assisting countries any country to deal with its health financing challenges, but economic growth political commitment, strategic intent, and astute management, are key ingredients, and as we would argue in this discussion, healthcare ICT, the underlying unifier and enabler. There is no doubt that many of the diseases responsible for the seemingly relentless increase in healthcare spending are preventable. The question is whether we are doing enough to prevent them. Until May 18, 2006 when the World Health Organization (WHO) confirmed details of a large cluster of human cases of H5N1 avian flu in Indonesia, heightening fears regarding human-to-human transmission of the virus and with questions asked about the role of genetic diathesis in why some people exposed to the virus become infected and others do not, did complacency reign? That H5N1 does not hop to humans from birds more frequently, considering the large numbers of exposures of individuals to infected poultry in some countries, makes this question even more pertinent. However, confirmation of the deaths in the village of Kubu Sembilang in the Karo district of North Sumatra of six members of one family who had reportedly contracted the virus no doubt suggests genetic vulnerability of this family compared to other families, and that we could no longer be complacent about human-to-human transmission of the virus. Indeed, on May 27, 2006, WHO placed the Swiss manufacturer of Tamiflu, Roche Holding AG on alert to get ready for the global stockpile of the anti-viral drug, the company in fact has already given WHO five million courses of treatment, and with the assistance of global partners, would produce 400 million courses a year by 2007. WHO officials have confirmed 36 deaths from bird flu in Indonesia, and reported 124 globally since late 2003. The Indonesian family cluster is the largest seen to date, but others previously occurred in Turkey and Azerbaijan. Also troubling are the chances of clusters of cases signaling what we have all anticipated with much trepidation, that of human-to-human transmission of the virus. So, has the virus mutated and is now able to jump form one person to another, or is the cluster mentioned above simply bird to human transmission in a genetically predisposed family? Either way, we need to act and fast. Human-to-human transmission of H5N1 could mean an imminent pandemic. The presence of a genetic diathesis means we need to know how prevalent it is, and if the virus had anything to do with its expression. These recent developments show that we must not be complacent about these issues, and call for actions that are even more urgent and programs to prevent a pandemic, and prepare for one if it happened such as developing and distributing vaccines and medications. There is also no doubt about the need to intensify research efforts to establish the presence or otherwise of genetic vulnerability to the virus, which would involve ruling out shared exposures, conditions, and habits, and other confounding factors. Even if we could not change the genetic makeup of persons now, we could perhaps develop a simple test that could identify those with this vulnerability, and take extra measures to protect them from the virus. We could for example, using a variety of multi-media healthcare ICT suited to the cultural milieu, and deployed within available technical infrastructure, disseminate not only information requesting testing for the diathesis but also on practices to adopt or avoid in other to prevent the expression of the disease. Perhaps we could do something about the virus interacting with these individuals' genes to express their vulnerability in disease, for example, developing a drug that interferes with the processes involved in such expression. The point is that H5N1 remains a major menace to humans and we have to act now to stop the virus. Here is one example that tests the core of our commitment to our disease prevention paradigm, because and as the World Bank report mentioned earlier emphasized, it reveals the multi-level dimensions of the Millennium Development Goals and how much more we need to do as a global community in achieving them. In other words, we need to conceptualize prevention at different yet intercalated levels, from the individual, to the local, national, and global levels, lack of action in one spilling over and eventually compromising the others, and the entire global health, and by extension, economic systems. Put differently, we need to start conceptualizing health as what could make or break our world, as we know it, and the prevention paradigm, as our best chance of fostering the former, and averting the latter. Viewed from its primary, secondary, and tertiary perspectives, our efforts become more focused, and our chances of achieving our goals, much higher. That we could achieve many of these prevention efforts deploying cost-effective healthcare ICT, even in developing countries, yet as some experts argue, the adoption of these technologies in the health industry lags behind other information-intensive industries such as the banking industry by as much as a decade, speaks volume to the need for change. Change in the health industry, that is. Embracing the prevention paradigm is the key towards making and effecting the changes necessary in the health industry to prevent the possible devastating consequences for the future of humankind that not so doing could engender. Yet again, merely appreciating the need for prevention is not enough, we must take the next logical step, which is to act on the paradigm. Such actions must aim at yielding positive results in the most efficient and cost-effective manner. In other words, they need to take our current limitations in resources into account, and not plunge us into economic chaos. In short, we must aim to achieve the dual objectives of delivering qualitative and effective health services simultaneously reducing health costs. Here is where the need for widespread healthcare ICT diffusion comes in, as these technologies could no doubt help improve the processes and reduce the transaction costs involved in health services delivery, and there is increasing research evidence to support this assertion at all levels of the prevention paradigm.

Research studies have shown, for example the benefits of media-based behavioral treatments for children with behavioral problems[1]. The treatment of behavioral problems in children is via a variety of approaches including medication or, more typically, psychological treatments with the child and/or family members. Behavioral and cognitive-behavioral interventions are highly effective but their usually long durations and cost issues have often restricted access to this treatment modality. A recent review, by researchers at the Centre for Evidence-Based Social Work, University of Oxford, examined the effects of media-based cognitive-behavioral therapies for any young person with a behavioral disorder, diagnosed using a valid instrument, versus standard care and no-treatment controls. The researchers wanted to know if giving parents the information they need in order to manage these behavior problems in media-based format would reduce the cost and increase access to these treatments using data and information obtained from an extensive search of a variety of databases. The searches were for randomized and quasi-randomized controlled trials of media-based behavioral treatments for behavior problems in children. The researchers included 11 studies, and 943 participants in the review, and found that in general, media-based therapies for behavioral disorders in children had a moderate, albeit variable, effect when compared with both no-treatment controls, with significant improvements made adding up to two hours of therapist time. They concluded that delivering behavioral interventions for carers of children via media formats might not just be sufficient to change a child's behavior significantly, in some cases, but also cut down how much time primary care workers offer each child. We could also use this approach as the preliminary stage of a stepped care approach. The approach would increase the number of families that could benefit from these treatments, freeing up physician's time for use in other tasks. In short, these media-based therapies offer both clinical and economic advantages regarding the treatment of children with behavioral problems. Many other studies have demonstrated the potential of healthcare ICT in enabling us achieve the dual objectives mentioned earlier. It is up to us to embrace, implement, and use these technologies and to promote their widespread diffusion among all healthcare stakeholders pursuant to our intention to achieve our healthcare delivery goals, which is beginning to seem like a survival imperative, if not in fact, one out of which we could no longer wriggle. Consider the findings of a recent study on diabetes, in the U.S for example that showed that a third of adults in the country do not even know, that they have the disease. There has been an increase in the prevalence of diagnosed diabetes in U.S. adults age 20 years and older from about 5.1% to 6.5%, noted researchers at the National Institutes of Health (NIH) and the Centers for Disease Control and Prevention (CDC), on analyzing national survey data from 2 periods, 1988 to 1994, and 1999 to 2002. Nonetheless, the figures for adults with undiagnosed diabetes remained relatively stable during the same period, and about 2.8% adults, one-third of persons with diabetes, still do not know that they have it. According to the study, published in the June 2006 issue of *Diabetes Care*, type 2 diabetes comprises about 95% of all diabetes cases, and almost all undiagnosed diabetes cases. The researchers found about 26% of adults age 20 years and older had persistent impaired fasting glucose (IFG), a form of pre-diabetes. IFG, when blood glucose measured after an overnight fast is high (100 to 125 milligrams per deciliter or mg/dL) but not high enough to be diagnostic of diabetes, and not only predisposes an individual to developing type 2 diabetes, but also heart disease. According to Dr. Larry Blonde, chair of the National Diabetes Education Program (NDEP), which the NIH, CDC, and 200 partner-organizations cosponsored, "It's important to know if you have pre-diabetes or undiagnosed type 2 Diabetes". He added, "You should talk to your health care professional about your risk. If your blood glucose is high but not high enough to be diagnosed as diabetes, losing weight and increasing physical activity will greatly lower your risk of getting type 2 diabetes. If you have diabetes, controlling your blood glucose, blood pressure, and cholesterol will prevent or delay the complications of diabetes." Considering that diabetes is the commonest cause of blindness, kidney failure, and amputations in adults and a significant cause of heart disease and stroke, should we not be doing whatever we could to alert the public to latent and manifest diabetes? Could healthcare ICT not help in so doing, and indeed, in implementing targeted and contextualized health information dissemination on this subject? Among other findings by the researchers are that almost 22% of people aged 65 years and older had diabetes. Does this not speak to the need for us to intensify secondary and tertiary prevention programs among our seniors to reduce morbidities and mortalities due to this disease, and would the use of appropriate healthcare ICT not help in achieving this objective cost-effectively, for example monitoring and controlling their blood sugar at home? What are the implications for resource allocation and utilization of the findings in the study that about 13% of non-Hispanic, blacks age 20 and older had diabetes that the condition was twice as common in non-Hispanic blacks compared to non-Hispanic whites and that about 8% of Mexican Americans age 20 and older had diabetes? After adjusting for age and sex, which makes the average age of Mexican Americans younger than for other groups, the researchers found that the prevalence of diabetes in Mexican Americans was twice that of non-Hispanic whites and about equal to that of non-Hispanic blacks. Do these figures not support the need for such targeted and contextualized health information mentioned earlier, and would this approach not apply in general to ensuring the effectiveness of health education and disease prevention campaigns in other multicultural countries such as Canada and the U.K? What are the implications for healthcare costs of the findings in the study that IFG and undiagnosed diabetes were about 70% commoner in men than in women, especially in non-Hispanic white men, and that almost 40% of people aged 65 years and older had IFG its prevalence in fact increasing with age? Should we not be doing something urgently to reduce these statistics if we were serious about reducing healthcare costs, for example intensifying our prevention strategies at all levels, which more widespread diffusion of healthcare ICT could help us achieve? Would it not be cheaper for those at risk for example to have the necessary health information on the disease than wait for them to seek this information, considering the difficulties obtaining accurate and current information on health conveniently? We should indeed pay more attention to this concept of healthcare ICT-enabled, targeted health information as it could significantly increase awareness and reduce the prevalence of this and other diseases, acute, and chronic, and in particular the latter, which are the chief healthcare cost drivers in contemporary healthcare delivery particularly in the developed countries. As we noted earlier, appropriately deployed in secondary and tertiary prevention, these technologies could also help reduce the rate and duration of hospitalizations, and the use of prescription medications, thus substantially reducing healthcare costs as they would, morbidities and mortalities, which among our seniors who often have a variety of other illnesses, could significantly reduce disease burden. According to lead-author Catherine Cowie, Ph.D., of the National Institute of Diabetes and Digestive and Kidney Diseases (NIDDK), "We're seeing a rising prevalence of diagnosed diabetes that is not substantially offset by a drop in the rate of undiagnosed, about one-third of adults with diabetes still don't know they have it. Another 26% of adults have a form of pre-diabetes." Would it not help to increase awareness of the danger lurking behind pre-diabetes, which typically causes no symptoms, for example that with the condition undiagnosed and nothing done about if diagnosed, many persons that have it would within a decade develop type 2 diabetes, and possibly also a heart attack or stroke even if type 2 diabetes does not emerge? Would persons with pre-diabetes knowing that they could prevent or delay diabetes if they lost a modest amount of weight by reducing their calorie intake and by being more active physically, such as walking 30 minutes a day 5 days a week not help stimulate interest in carrying out these simple measures? One key study of individuals with impaired glucose tolerance (IGT), when blood glucose levels are high two hours after a sugary drink, but not high enough for diagnosing diabetes, showed that lifestyle changes resulting in a 5 to 7% weight loss reduced diabetes onset by 58%. Should our efforts to inform the public about these measures not be more vigorous? Experts recommend that persons over 45 years old should consult their doctors about testing for pre-diabetes or diabetes, and if younger, overweight, and have another risk factor, also do the same. Should we not let this information out, and in fact alert the public to the risk factors for pre-diabetes and type 2 diabetes such as being 45 years or older, with a family history of diabetes, overweight, and not physically active, for example exercise less than three times a week? Other risk factors are belonging to a high-risk ethnic population such as being African American, Hispanic/Latino American, American Indian and Alaska Native, Asian American, and a Pacific Islander. Individuals with high blood pressure: 140/90 mm/Hg or higher, who have an HDL cholesterol less than 35 mg/dL or a triglyceride level 250 mg/dL or higher, have had diabetes that developed during pregnancy (gestational Diabetes) or have given birth to a baby weighing more than 9 pounds, are at risk. Those that have polycystic ovary syndrome, which is a metabolic disorder affecting the female reproductive system are also at risk. So are those that have acanthosis nigricans, which is a dark, thickened skin around neck or armpits, have a history of disease of the blood vessels to the heart, brain, or legs, or have had IFG or IGT on previous testing. On April 25, the National Diabetes Education Program (NDEP) launched a new diabetes prevention message: *It's Never Too Early to Prevent Diabetes. A Lifetime of Small Steps for a Healthy Family*, the sort of collaborative prevention effort more of which we should initiate not just in the U.S but in other countries too. About 2 million Canadians have diabetes, which costs the country $9 billion yearly, the condition three to five times more prevalent among Aboriginal people. Ohinmaa et. al in a study published in vol. 28 of the Canadian Journal of Diabetes projected the prevalence and cost of diabetes mellitus in Canada and its provinces for the years 2000 to 2016[2]. The authors stated that the number of persons with diabetes in the general population in Canada would increase from about 1.4 million patients in 2000 to 2.4 million patients in 2016, and estimated the total healthcare costs to increase from C$4.66 billion in 2000 to $8.14 billion in 2016 (1996 dollar values). The authors also noted that if the current trends continued, both the number of individuals with diabetes and healthcare costs, would increase by over 70% during the same period, with a 12% increase in projected overall population and about 72% projected increase in the prevalence of diabetes. The authors projected these changes would be highest in the provinces with the highest population increases and the most rapid population aging. They acknowledged that the projections could not fully account for changes in management strategies for diabetes and comorbidities and complications of diabetes. Thus, the widespread implementation and use of cost-saving healthcare ICT could result in overestimation of total healthcare costs in this study, or underestimation were seniors to live longer with more efficient dialysis, for example. Could we not aim at reducing costs using cost-effective and efficient healthcare ICT in primary prevention initiatives, and in assertively in secondary and tertiary prevention obviating the need for costly hospitalizations? A 2005 study, the Diabetes in Canada

Evaluation (DICE) study, the largest diabetes study of its nature in Canada, showed that only one in two Canadians had their diabetes well controlled. The Canadian government in 1999 allotted $115 million to the Canadian Diabetes Strategy (CDS) to combat the disease, via primary, secondary, and tertiary prevention programs. In Ontario, which has 800,000 persons that have diabetes, and another 200,000 in whom it might be latent, government earmarked $68 million to support Chronic Disease Prevention and Health Promotion programs and services in 2006, with $8 million in additional funding allocated in the 2006 budget to increase physical activity participation in the province. These measures would, no doubt help reduce the risk of type 2 diabetes and its associated costs. The government also committed $12 million to insulin pumps and supplies for children, which would help 6,500 children with type 1 diabetes to better manage their condition, and boost both the efforts regarding secondary and tertiary prevention, of complications such heart and kidney diseases, and possible loss of vision. There are over 1 million persons with diabetes in the UK, the number expected to increase to 3 million by 2010, and another well over a million people that have the condition but are unaware that they do. Estimates of the exact cost of diabetes vary. However, according to one study, the disease constituted about 9% of the annual NHS budget [3], roughly £5.2 billion a year. In the U.K, up to 10% of hospital budgets is spent on treating diabetes and its complications, NHS spending on diabetes will rise to 10% by 2011, persons with diabetes spend 1.1 million days annually in hospital and £500 million of their own money on coping with the disease, the Social Services costs, about £230 million. It cost the NHS up to £30 million a year to treat new cases of diabetic kidney failure. Indeed, the British Diabetic Association (BDA) is calling for the routine screening of many more seniors for type-2 diabetes, which on average, remains undiagnosed for seven years, by which time complications have already set in. Does this not support the need for healthcare ICT-enabled prevention measures that even seniors could use at home to screen, monitor, and manage their blood sugar, connected to their doctor's electronic medical record (EMR) systems for supervision and management? The BDA anticipates the number of type-2 diabetics to increase in the future, due to increasing overweight/obesity, and an ageing population. In Australia, estimated health spending on diabetes in 2000‾01 was around $784 million, 1.7% of allocatable recurrent health expenditure, diabetes thus 15th of about 200 disease groups evaluated, $204 million spent on antidiabetic drugs and diabetes testing reagents. Only 10% of the 4.6 million prescriptions for antidiabetic drugs in the same period were for insulin, yet they accounted for 60% of expenditure on antidiabetic drugs. In Europe, the Costs of Diabetes in Europe - Type 2 survey (CODE-2) examined thousands of patients in eight countries, and found that only 2.7% of the total health spending on diabetes was on oral medication to control the disease, hospitalization costs and for complications of the disease, 30%, and 65% of the total spending. The costs of medications to treat long-term complications and as "second-line" treatments once oral medication became ineffective were between 18% and 39% of costs, depending on the country surveyed. Overall, healthcare spending on persons with diabetes accounted for 5% of the total healthcare expenditure of each country. Do these figures not underscore the need for us to put more effort into our prevention efforts, particularly at the primary level? Do they not in fact highlight the need to seek more cost-effective ways to address the problems relating to this disease, and indeed other chronic diseases, particularly among our seniors, who have most from these diseases? Should we not intensify our efforts to promote the widespread diffusion of healthcare ICT, technologies that if appropriately deployed could help us achieve the dual goals of qualitative healthcare delivery while reducing costs? Would these technologies for example not help improve access to healthcare for individuals that either would or already have developed these preventable diseases? In the U.S., over 45 million do not have health insurance. These individuals lack or potentially lack access to health services. They fall into different income levels, those in the lower income brackets some studies indicate, would likely use fewer recommended health services than those in the higher income brackets, but is this so? A recent study published in the May 3, 2006 issue of the Journal of the American Medical Association[4], provides us with the answer to this question. The researchers found the use of cancer prevention services by eligible adults to range from 51% to 88% for colorectal and cervical cancer screening, respectively. They found the range for the use of cardiovascular risk reduction services to be from 38% to 81%, for weight loss counseling, and aspirin use, respectively, that for the use of services for diabetes management, from 33% to 88% for pneumococcal vaccination and serum glycosylated-hemoglobin measurement respectively. They also noted the strong link of health insurance and annual household income with use of almost all the health care services they looked at. Findings from this study also showed no significant increase in the likelihood of uninsured versus insured adults receiving recommended health care services for cancer prevention, cardiovascular risk reduction, or diabetes management due to higher annual household incomes. In other words, there is a significant link between lack of health care insurance and decreased use of recommended health care services even among higher-income adults, just as there is among lower-income adults. The researchers recommended attention to patient education, and expanding insurance eligibility for both categories of individuals in our efforts to improve the use of recommended health care services. This study highlights some of the issues germane to addressing the challenges that contemporary healthcare delivery confront, namely, delivering qualitative healthcare while simultaneously reducing the ever-increasing health spending in many countries, particularly in the developed world. Could we for example in the U.S. say that we are delivering such services with even persons in the higher-income brackets not receiving the care that they need because they lack health insurance? What could the ramifications of this be for the burden of disease on the individuals, their families, and on society? Considering that, these individuals are not utilizing the services that could prevent the diseases that constitute significant drivers of healthcare spending does this problem not warrant urgent focus, to find the appropriate solutions to the problem? Is it any wonder for example that the Centers for Medicare and Medicaid(CMS) Administrator Mark McClellan on May 19, 2006 announced at a luncheon that the Galen Institute and the Council for Affordable Health Insurance co-sponsored that it plans to increase the use of preventive services among Medicare beneficiaries to help "close the prevention gap,"? Medicare currently offers preventive services such as an initial physical for new beneficiaries, cardiovascular tests, cancer screenings, and flu vaccinations. The Administrator noted that CMS has started to track the use of preventive services among Medicare beneficiaries to make certain that those that need such services receive them, and that CMS would collaborate with community groups across the country to increase awareness about the preventive services Medicare provides. McClellan also hinted that Medicare would likely include health savings accounts (HSAs) in its coverage options for beneficiaries in 2007. The focus on prevention by CMS is not only desirable, but also necessary, considering the gains in health status improvement and in costs savings that could accrue from these efforts. Let us examine the recent findings of a long-term study of middle-aged women that showed that women who do not have enough shut-eye each night risk gaining weight, presented on May 24, 2006 by a Cleveland-based researcher reported at the American Thoracic Society's International Conference in San Diego, California. Women that slept 5 hours or less each night were 32% more likely to gain a significant amount of weight, 33 pounds or more, and 15% more likely to become obese than women who slept 7 hours each night. The study also showed that women who slept 6 hours every night were 12% likelier to gain weight and 6% likelier to become obese versus those that slept 7 hours every night. On the average, women that slept for 5 hours or less each night weighed 5.4 pounds more at the start of the study than those that slept for 7 hours. The study followed the 68,183 participants up for 16 years. The study also found that with the effect of age and weight at the start of the study eliminated, women that slept 5 hours or less, and those that slept 6 hours each night gained roughly 2.3 pounds and 1.5 pounds more respectively on follow-up than those who slept 7 hours ever night. Not even differences in diet and physical activity levels of the women influenced the findings, and in fact, the researchers found that women that slept less ate less. With regard exercise, the findings revealed a small difference in that women who slept less exercised slightly less than women who slept more, but this did not fully explain the other findings. The authors concluded that less sleep may affect changes in basal metabolic rate, the number of calories one burns at rest, or may be individuals that sleep less also have less "non-exercise associated thermogenesis' or NEAT, that is, involuntary activity such as fidgeting or standing rather than sitting, in other words, fidget less. A weight gain of 33 pounds (15kg.) unquestionable increases the risk for developing diabetes and heart disease, two of the commonest diseases that become chronic, are relatively common in seniors, and are significant healthcare costs drivers. How could the findings of this study help those of our women that need to or want to lose weight accomplish this goal? Should we not let our women know about the findings in this study? Could the high prevalence of sleep problems in the U.S have any bearing on the equally high prevalence of overweight/obesity in the country, and if so, should we not refocus our efforts on helping people, particularly women to sleep better and longer? Would this not help improve their overall health status, reduce the prevalence of chronic diseases due to excessive weight, and reduce health spending overall? Could some women provided the findings of this study not seek other ways to lose weight than smoke cigarettes for example, the reason many give for picking up or sustaining the habit? Do these questions not speak to the need for targeted and contextualized health information dissemination, being a key aspect of our efforts to implement our disease prevention paradigm? Do they not also reassure us that implementing the paradigm would help us achieve the dual objectives of providing all with qualitative healthcare while reducing health spending simultaneously?

Overweight/obesity causes a variety of other health problems, including, according

to a study published in the May 22, 2006 issue of *Cancer*, increasing the overall risk of breast cancer in women. The study, which noted that the women who gain weight as adults have a higher lifetime risk of all types of breast cancer, further support current evidence of the link between weight and breast cancer. Over 44,000 women participated in the study that found that the more weight a woman gained, the higher the risk for all types, stages, and grades of breast cancer she faces. A gain in weight of over 60pounds (27kg) about doubles a woman's risk of developing ductal type breast tumors and increases by over 1.5 times her likelihood of developing lobular type cancers versus another that gained 20 pounds (10 kg) or less during adulthood. The researchers also found that the risk of breast cancer that had spread tripled for women with over 60 pounds (27 kg) weight gain. That fat tissue produces estrogen compounds the risk of breast cancer, already linked to increased estrogen levels. Do these findings not underscore the need for women to maintain a healthy body weight throughout adulthood? With breast cancer being the number two leading cause of cancer death among U.S. women, second only to lung cancer, and over 200,000 people diagnosed and another approximately 40,000 die from breast cancer annually, and over 1.2 million men and women developing breast cancer every year, is this not a major public health issue? Should women not know about the link of breast cancer to weight, the latter they could readily control successfully in a variety of ways? Another study published in May 2006 noted that women who take estrogen-only hormone replacement therapy for two decades or more, to treat symptoms of menopause have an increased risk of developing breast cancer. Should women also not know about this important finding? Is the prospect of being able to prevent these diseases in women by simply getting the word out regarding the findings of these studies not going to be cost-effective? There is no doubt that the answer many would give to this question would be in the affirmative, but how should we get women to know about these findings, wait for them to seek health information, or deliver it to them? The rate at which new medical knowledge emerges is simply to fast for even healthcare professionals to keep track. Many therefore miss important findings that they could pass on to their patients or incorporate into their practice to improve healthcare delivery to their patients. This is not only a disservice to the immense efforts of medical and other researchers, and the immense financial and other resources invested in these efforts, but it also perpetrates the pernicious information asymmetry that plagues the healthcare industry. How could we avail ourselves of the rich and veritable information these researches produce with the information buried in an avalanche of data that confront us routinely? How could a healthcare consumer be discerning in the choice of service provision, including medications, and lab investigations, lacking the vital information required to make rational choices on these issues? Despite the increasing ubiquity of the Internet for example, and the ease and availability of Internet search engines, cancer patients seeking information about their disease found more via a librarian than by searching on their own. This finding emerged from a new study from the University of Michigan Comprehensive Cancer Center presented at the May 21, 2006, annual meeting of the Medical Library Association. The researchers surveyed patients and families visiting the Cancer Center's Patient Education Resource Center (PERC) regarding the information they obtained subsequent to a search request. Sixty five percent of visitors said that the professional search returned information they did not obtain from other sources, another 30% that the librarian even offered new information, with just 4% saying they found information on their own. Does this study not attest to the need for targeted health information dissemination? Would there not be others seeking health information who could not go to a library, and would not find Internet search engines useful, either because they returned a load of information that sifting through would be an unwelcome chore or, indeed, of irrelevant information.? Many individuals are no doubt unaccustomed to search strategies and techniques that are critical to finding the information one needs via search engines, but trying to find specific health information could be frustrating for others, and result in these latter folks giving up and not trying again to find the information that they need. Should we not be doing something to prevent this sort of frustration if we were serious about achieving the dual objectives of reducing healthcare costs without compromising the quality of service delivery? Participants in this study no doubt found the expertise of librarians in searching useful. Should we not provide the health consumer with this expertise in their living rooms, particularly as not everyone would be able to visit the library, nor is it realistic to expect people to do so in order to seek every piece of health information that they need. There would of course be individuals who, seeking an in-depth knowledge of their illnesses, or who need answers to questions on vexing medical issues and new discoveries in medications, and surgical procedures, for example, would consult a professional librarian. However, many in the developed world would attempt to obtain this information via the Internet. Again, there are web sites that have credible health information, but most carry basic, outdated, hence probably inaccurate, sometimes even deliberately skewed information that could prove more harmful than helpful to the healthcare consumer. Rectifying the information asymmetry in healthcare that these problems and others engender is a vital task in our efforts to achieve the dual objectives mentioned above. Consider also a recent, randomized controlled trial presented at the May 4, 2006, annual scientific meeting of the American Geriatrics Society (AGS,), a study that showed that breaking off the pathway between depression and death, closely linked in the elderly, could improve survival of the seniors significantly. The trial based on data from the randomized, multisite Prevention of Suicide in Primary Care Elderly: Collaborative Trial (PROSPECT), between 1999 and 2003, looked at an intervention to treat depression in seniors in primary care. The researchers assumed that depression is a risk factor for death, chances for modifying which risk via intervention, there was hitherto a dearth of research, and which chances they sought to analyze. The researchers found that depressed patients in practices that provided depression care management were less likely to expire during a 4-year period than were depressed patients in usual-care practices, hence concluded that besides reducing morbidity, which we already know, depression care management in primary care, could also reduce mortality, which this study first revealed. It is not only desirable for our seniors to live for as long and as qualitatively as possible, which should be the goal of healthcare delivery to them, in fact, the longer they live, the less end-of-life healthcare costs they incur. Researches have shown that younger seniors tend to incur more end-of-life costs due to the types and nature of the diseases they have, such as cardiovascular events in the heart and the brain, compared to older seniors in their eighties and nineties who often die of less expensive illnesses such as pneumonia. Should we then not get the word out both to family doctors and to seniors and their families of the dual benefits of reducing morbidity and mortality, treating depression in seniors? Should we perhaps not be preventing it in the first place, for example, by minimizing their isolation, loneliness, which many seniors experience after losing their spouses, siblings, and friends, being a prime factor in plunging them into depression? The studies we have discussed so far not only illustrate the need for health information dissemination, preferably targeted, which deploying the appropriate healthcare ICT could help achieve efficiently and cost-effectively, but also the importance of such information dissemination for different levels of the disease prevention paradigm. Thus healthcare ICT-backed targeted health information dissemination would enable us achieve our primary, secondary, and tertiary prevention goals. Essentially primary prevention is preventing the disease from occurring in the first place, secondary, its prompt diagnosis and treatment, and tertiary, the prevention of its sequelae. With seniors being the most ardent healthcare consumer, hence on whom we expend a significant portion of health dollars we cannot possibly gainsay the need to redouble our efforts on focusing on the role that ICT could play in actualizing our disease prevention initiatives. Recent developments on Capitol Hill lend credence to this statement.

On May 25, 2006, the House Ways and Means Subcommittee on Health in the U.S

voted 8-5 to approve a bill, HR4157, which would promote the use of healthcare ICT and create national standards on privacy and implementation of electronic health records (EHR). Subcommittee Chair Nancy Johnson (R-Conn.) and Rep. Nathan Deal (R-Ga.) co-sponsored the legislation. Further, the law would codify the Office of the National Coordinator for Health Information Technology within the Department of Health Human Services (HHS). Its goals also include creating a committee that would advice on national standards for medical data storage and develop a permanent structure for national interoperability standards governance. The bill also has provisions for medical privacy laws including ensuring that current laws apply to data stored or transmitted electronically and oblige the HHS secretary to suggest to Congress a privacy standard that could harmonize federal and state laws. The bill also provides for an increase in the number of billing codes health care providers use to file insurance claims from 24,000 to over 200,000 by Oct. 1, 2009. We all should applaud a Bill such as this and other countries should indeed, pass similar bills, considering the importance of these technologies in facilitating the achievement our dual healthcare delivery objectives. A recent Quebec study on the benefits of having pictures of the pathological effects of cigarette smoking on cigarettes, which is ongoing in Canada, as part of the efforts to discourage cigarette smoking, showed that these pictures did not discourage chronic smokers, but did persons that had not at all started to smoke. Should we not explore other means, perhaps via innovative healthcare ICT, by which we could develop more contextualized and effective prevention programs for chronic smokers? Would such a program not require the widespread use of these technologies that the Bill mentioned above could help achieve? In fact, should we not also devise such contextualized healthcare ICT-backed preventive programs targeted at young people, and by promoting the technologies that could actualize such programs are we not investing in the future health of our youngsters, who would not only grow in healthier adults, but also healthier seniors? Consider a recent 2000-pupil study in Tobacco Control, which Cancer Research UK sponsored, and which indicated that children who try just one cigarette are twice as likely to commence smoking as those who have never tried it, even after a break of three years or more. The study points to a sort of "sleeper effect" of cigarette smoking, with the interest in the habit persisting years after the first cigarette, even if only just one, which prompted Cancer Research UK to recommend that anti-smoking campaigns target stopping children from smoking any cigarette at all, even one. The link between cigarette smoking and a variety of lung diseases such as chronic bronchitis, emphysema, even lung cancer, is no longer in doubt, nor is the burden of these disease in human and material terms. Healthcare ICT offers us options in targeted health information delivery to this tech-savvy population segment, which we should exploit maximally. However, we need to promote the use of these technologies by healthcare organizations in both the private and public sectors, and indeed, by other interested healthcare stakeholders, for example, advocacy groups, in initiating contextualized campaigns that would further reinforce the dangers of cigarette. The study mentioned earlier for example, which surveyed young people in 36 London schools annually from 11years to 16years, found that about 14% of 11-year olds and 62% of 15-year olds have smoked a cigarette, hence the researchers' recommendation that we should start such targeted prevention initiatives at children while they are still at primary school. The study found that the 12% of 11-12 year olds who said that they smoked only once were more likely to commence smoking when older versus those who had never smoked, even after a 3-year lull. According to Dr Jennifer Fidler, study leader and a research psychologist at the Cancer Research UK Health Behavior Unit in London, it is the first study that shows an early experience with one cigarette, leads to smoking several years later. The researchers noted that this "sleeper effect" could be because nicotine in a single cigarette may influence brain pathways thereby increasing one's prospects of picking up smoking subsequent to other cues such as stress, or that first trial might dissolve prior inhibitory barriers on smoking, for example getting caught, or concern on how to smoke. According to Dr Jennifer Fidler, "It is known that past smoking behavior predicts future behavior and it could take some time to progress from an experimental to regular smoker"·'But this is the first study that shows an early experience with one cigarette leads to smoking several years in the future". She also noted that "There are two important messages - firstly it may be more important than previously thought to try and prevent children from trying even one cigarette and, secondly, health professionals and those working in smoking prevention in schools need to be aware that those who have tried one cigarette, but are not smokers, are at risk." This study also raises the question whether even one cigarette might have an addictive effect, particularly as previous researches have indicated that there is conditioning of nicotine receptors, even with second-hand smoke, as children of parents that smoke in the youngsters' presence are likelier to smoke. Should we therefore, not encourage the adoption of healthcare ICT, which could help facilitate these prevention efforts, by healthcare professionals, and others that might be involved in creating and implementing the necessary health-education campaign programs? In the U.K., the Department of Health is taking new steps to deter smokers, requesting public opinion on a series of picture warnings to appear on and cover 40% of the back of cigarette packets from autumn 2007. Members of the public could give their opinion on a number of images designed to highlight the dangers of smoking on a specified website. They could also choose images to support 14 health messages such as "Smoking causes fatal lung cancer" or "Smoking may reduce blood flow and causes impotence". This measure takes stark written warnings already on cigarette packs sold in the country a step further, but as noted earlier with the Quebec study, even if it did not deter chronic smokers, it probably would, youngsters, from taking up the habit, which is just as crucial an objective to aim for. Besides, evidence from Brazil and elsewhere, showed that the approach not only informed people of the risks of smoking, and deglamorise it, but also helped encourage them to reduce or quit smoking. Many welcome the measure, even suggested that the messages should be at the front, and not the back of the cigarette packs. Others oppose singling out smokers arguing there should be such graphic warnings against fatty foods, dairy products, alcohol, and other products with adverse health effects. There is no doubt about the need to address the health issues of a variety of products, and take the necessary prevention measures to combat those that are adverse, and employing targeted, multimedia, contextualized, healthcare ICT-enabled health information dissemination is no doubt one of the most efficient and cost-effective ways to achieve this goal. Thus, for example, we do not even want our children to discover the health hazards of cigarette smoking only after they have decided to buy a pack. It might simply be too late to stop many, hence the need for additional targeted health information delivered to young people that would discourage them from even contemplating buying the cigarette in the first place, particular in view of the "sleeper effect" mentioned above. In fact, even among adults, with reference to preventing the adverse consequences of cigarette smoking on health, these efforts take different dimensions, including legislating against the habit, as the example of Ontario's new anti-smoking legislation, set to take effect on June 01, 2006, shows. The Smoke-Free Ontario Act, reputedly one of the toughest in North America, outlaws smoking in enclosed public spaces and all workplaces, such as bars, restaurants, casinos, and bingo halls. Further, by June 2008, the law mandates retailers to remove their self-styled cigarette "power walls" and replace them with a new display where minors cannot see them. Despite opposition from affected businesses and others, provincial politicians and health officials insist that the smoking laws will reduce the health-care costs linked with smoking-related diseases, prevent youngsters from starting to smoke, and help smokers to relinquish the habit. Ninety six percent of Ontario residents support smoking restrictions, and 67% considered the legislation would pressure smokers to stop smoking, according to a recent survey. In early May 2006, Ontario Health Promotion Minister Jim Watson actually announced an extra $5.5 million for public health units to help pay for the over 100 enforcement officers that would ensure compliance with the law. It is hardly surprising that Ontario has taken this step to prevent the perpetration of the adverse consequences of cigarette smoking on the health of its residents, forty four of whom die daily from tobacco-related diseases, its number one preventable cause of death. To be sure, 80% of the province's residents do not smoke, and tobacco consumption rates fell almost 10% in Ontario in the past year, but the government envisages that the new law would further reduce this figure, by 20% in 2007. As earlier noted, our prevention efforts could be along any of three dimensions, namely, primary, secondary, and tertiary, and our goals should not be simply to formulate programs for each, but also to implement them, and indeed, to do so in the most efficient and cost-effective manner. Thus, healthcare ICT appropriately deployed could facilitate not only Ontario residents, but in particular the businesses that the new anti-smoking law mentioned above, knowing about the law, but also how the benefits derivable from it far outweigh the costs, even if in the long term. Such campaigns would help improve its acceptance and compliance to the law, perhaps even reduce the need for, hence the costs of enforcement. These issues underscore the need to continue to promote the widespread adoption of healthcare ICT in healthcare delivery, and how these technologies could enable us achieve our objectives in this regard, more efficiently, and cost-effectively. Lack of access to care is one of the key issues hindering secondary prevention. How could we expect to diagnose and treat illnesses promptly when people do not have coverage to see the doctors and other healthcare professionals to perform these tasks? This is why the Bill that Iowa Republican Charles Grassley, chair of the Senate Finance Committee and an author of the 2003 Medicare drug law sponsored in the U.S Senate on May 16, 2006, which has bipartisan support, is apposite. The Bill would waive the penalty on

Americans who missed the May 16, 2006, deadline for Medicare drug coverage enrollment, who, about 1.5 million of Medicare's 42 million patients would have had to face a lifetime penalty. Until 2006, the federal health program for the elderly and disabled did not cover outpatient prescription drugs. Officials estimated that about 4.5 million would eventually be without drug coverage, roughly 3 million of who are low-income patients, who would receive penalties. There is no doubt that the benefit started on a difficult note for seniors in January 2006, problems mostly attributed to the unanticipated increases in the volume of information the computer systems involved in the operations had to cope with. This, again, underlines the need for not just implementing healthcare ICT, but making sure that the technologies perform their tasks efficiently, and cost-effectively. The said computer glitches would not only have compromised access by many seniors to their medications, which might have had adverse consequences for their health, and cost implications for Medicare, and other agencies involved in the plan. Thus, the need for the smooth running of implemented healthcare information systems in order to facilitate access to care, hence ensure that we achieve our secondary disease prevention objectives is indeed, urgent and crucial. This is also, why the Bill is not only apt but also fair, and important to promote the access to care that seniors crucially need. As Florida Democratic Sen. Bill Nelson, who had pushed unsuccessfully to get the May 15 deadline extended until the end of 2006, rightly put it, the new legislation "will give seniors more time to sign up without facing stiff financial penalties." If not waived, the penalty for anyone that signs up late is a lifetime surcharge of 1% of the monthly premium for the drug benefit monthly, and a 7% penalty for someone who missed the deadline, and then signed up in November 2006, the next chance to enroll, and even more for anyone who missed that. Few if any would dispute the importance of seniors gaining access to and receiving qualitative care without incurring expenses that they could hardly afford, and indeed, to encourage plans that enable the achievement of these goals. Some experts argue that this Bill would also help do just that by making up for a projected $1.7 billion in lost penalty revenue over five years reducing a "stabilization fund" meant to help private managed-care health plans care for seniors.

Healthcare ICT facilitates access to care but also improves other processes that together contribute to the efficient running of healthcare operations crucial to assuring the quality of healthcare delivery and saving costs. Thus, we need to promote the implementation of these technologies not only among healthcare professionals but also among other healthcare stakeholders, and there is evidence that this is starting to happen on a relatively large scale. America's Health Insurance Plans, a 150-member, trade group for the managed care industry, recently noted that a survey based on one week's transactions since Oct. 1, 2006, by each of its 26 insurance firms, revealed that 75% of current claims are now electronic, versus 44% four years ago. This attests to the increasing role of electronic claims-processing companies that help doctors and hospitals receive payment. That many hospitals, physicians, and pharmacies are now sending most of their bills to insurance firms digitally would no doubt help speed payment on claims an insurer did not reject, query, or delay, complete processing of 98% of accepted claims within 30 days of receipt for example, as the survey showed. It also showed a 1 in 7 claims rejection, returned to the doctor or hospital with the designation, "incomplete or incorrect". Virtually all pharmacies have submitted their claims digitally since the 1980's, and Medicare payments, excluded in the survey, require in the main, such electronic claims submission. The group also observed that delays sometimes emanated from the physician's end of the transaction, for example, 29% of claims arriving at the insurer over 30 days after patient treatment, which some doctors attributed to some insurers' demanding "difficult-to-collate" operating room notes or hospital records. However, this only further speaks to the need for automating data and information processing by healthcare providers. Would implementing electronic medical records (EMR), linked to regional health information networks (RHIN), for example, not prevent such delays by making it easy to gather, collate, and transmit information? Does this not also underscore the point about healthcare ICT diffusion in the health industry, with the information required for facilitating processes be they clinical, administrative, management and financial, available as and when needed, without any breach of confidentiality, as access would be graded, and specified, hence appropriately authenticated?

There is no doubt about the enormous costs of healthcare administration, not just in

the U.S, but also in many other countries. A study published in the August 21, 2003 issue of the New England Journal of Medicine (NEJM) noted that in 1993, the administrative costs of health care in the U.S far exceeded those in Canada, but that by 1999, they were at least $294.3 billion in the former or $1,059 per capita, versus $307 per capita in the latters. They arrived at the figures based on calculations of the administrative costs of health insurers, employers' health benefit programs, hospitals, practitioners' offices, nursing homes, and home care agencies, and excluded retail pharmacy sales and a few other categories for which they could not find relevant data. The authors also noted that upon exclusions, administration accounted for 31% of health care expenditures in the U.S., versus 16.7% in Canada, the overhead of whose national health insurance program was 1.3%, and among private insurers, 13.2% versus 11.7% in the U.S., although providers' administrative costs were much less in Canada. From 1969 to 1999, the share of the U.S. health care labor force that administrative workers accounted for increased from 18.2% to 27.3%, whereas it increased from 16.0% to 19.1% between 1971 and 1996 in Canada, for both countries, insurance-industry personnel excluded. The study concluded that the difference in what the U.S. and Canada spent on health care administration increased to $752 per capita, and that by implementing a Canadian-style health care system would help the U.S reduce these costs. To be sure, this study triggered a heated debate ranging from concerns about inaccurate statistics, biased analyses, and wrong conclusions. However, there was no contention over the fact that administrative costs are increasing in both countries. What's more, these are expenditures, money spent to provide or obtain goods or services, specific components and contributory to overall healthcare costs, costs defined as any outlay of resources may be money, labor, or time; or losses incurred because of a disease, or event, or lack of it. Expenditure therefore is a specific component of total costs. Costs due to diabetes for example would comprise among others, potential income lost, reduced quality of life (QOL), or years of life lost because of the disease and its complications of the to the effects of diabetes, and expenditure by persons, private firms, or governments on health services or medications. However, these costs might have been different, perhaps less because of shorter hospitalization or none at all, were the individual, say a senior, not lacking access to care due to administrative bottlenecks, for example as occurred with the introduction of the drug-benefit plan in January 2006. Even without clinical adverse consequences, it is only counterintuitive to allow administrative costs to get out of control, regardless of the type of healthcare system. Thus, this is a legitimate issue to address in effecting our prevention paradigm and ensuring its success. Lack of access to care goes counter to secondary prevention whose principle is essentially prompt diagnosis and treatment, and of course to tertiary prevention, which is preventing the onset of, or the worsening of the complications of a disease. It is therefore important for us to promote the use of healthcare ICT in non-clinical domains of the healthcare delivery systems as well. Thus, administration, and finance also ought to utilize these technologies to facilitate their processes and make them more effective and efficient. In fact, these arms of the health industry seem to have embraced health information systems for decades, although there is the need to improve continually, their legacy systems based on progress in these technologies, the need to comply with a variety of emerging legislation. For example, t he Administrative Simplification provisions of the Health Insurance Portability and Accountability Act of 1996 (HIPAA, Title II) oblige the Department of Health and Human Services (HHS) to institute national standards for electronic health care transactions and national identifiers for healthcare providers, health plans, and employers. The Act also deals with the security and privacy of health data. Indeed, according to the CMS, embracing these standards could only improve the efficiency and effectiveness of the country's healthcare system by promoting the pervasive employment of electronic data transactions in healthcare delivery. Another legitimate area of concern is regarding the depletion of available healthcare resources thereby making them unavailable for future use. One example is the use of prescription medications, which is a major cost driver in many health systems, particularly in the developed world. Besides, primary prevention would reduce the need for these prescriptions in the first place. On May 19, 2006, the largest pharmacy benefits manager in the U.S, Medco Health Solutions Inc., announced that it was distributing more generic than brand-name drugs, which was suggestive of pricey brand-name prescription medicines perhaps losing its market hold, with resulting reduced medications costs for the healthcare consumer. This development is even more significant considering the expectation of many more generic medications released to the market soon. There is no doubt that this would reduce healthcare costs for many, particularly, seniors, and individuals with chronic diseases. The company replaced 54% of drug prescriptions with generic equivalents, up from 47% in 2006. The company serves its 55 million members with health insurance, and distributes medications via mail or pharmacies through various prescription plans around the country. Because of the increasing use of generics in 2005, the firm was able to reduce the increase in prescription drug spending to its least increase rate in over five years, and drug spending increased 5.4% in 2005, versus 8.5% in 2004 and 16.4% in 1999. Although difficult to estimate, the increasing use of generics would likely contribute substantially to lowering healthcare costs, and to savings for individuals. According to CMS estimates, total health expenditures in 2006 would be $2.16 trillion, projected to increase to over $4 trillion in 2015. A key aspect of ensuring that healthcare consumers take the best decisions regarding their healthcare is for them to have the right information, at the right time, including on medications, hence the need to continue to promote the widespread diffusion of healthcare ICT, which could help to provide them with this information efficiently and cost-effectively. Such availability of health information would have played a role in health consumers knowing about the dangers of two widely used pain medications, Vioxx and Bextra, later withdrawn from the market, an action that also helped slowed prescription-drug spending in 2005. So did the caution by Food and Drugs Administration (FDA) of possible risk of heart disease due to the use of Celebrex, used to treat arthritis. There is no doubt about the shift toward the use of generics in preference to brands, as the health consumer becomes increasingly discerning particularly with more widespread implementation of healthcare ICT and their use rectifying the pervasive health information asymmetry in the health industry. The increasing demand by employers and other payers for the use of less costly medications and for lower healthcare in general would also help ensure this shift. To underscore this point, health plans, unions, and companies, have filed ten lawsuits over a tentative settlement that would delay the sale of a generic version of Plavix, the settlement, announced in March 2006, which would settle a patent infringement lawsuit that Sanofi-Aventis, and Bristol-Myers Squibb, which co-market the medication filed against generic pharmaceutical company Apotex. The settlement, which requires Federal Trade Commission endorsement, means that BMS and Sanofi would pay a certain amount to Apotex, which could start to market the generic version of Plavix in September 2011, eight months before the expiration of the U.S. patent. The ten lawsuits claim that the settlement would violate federal antitrust laws. The pharmaceutical industry is apparently bracing up for the huge changes the shift toward generics would bring to their operations, and strategic options. With many of the patents that gave the industry major boosts in the 1990s expiring in the next few years, the industry could not but expect these changes, particularly as such patent loss typically results 60% to 80% market share loss in the first year. This is what would likely happen in just four years to brand-name drugs, for examples, Ambien, Zoloft, and Zocor, among others with combined U.S. sales close to $43 billion. What is more, states are increasingly promulgating legislation permitting pharmacies to offer generics. Some would argue that increasing access to care is increasing healthcare costs. To some extent this is true, if the access to care is irrational and an abuse or misuse of the healthcare system. Furthermore, access to care does not always have to be to hospital care, with the individual incurring costs staying on hospital beds for weeks when he/she could have received treatment more cost-effectively and equally, if not more efficiently in an ambulatory/community/domiciliary setting. On the other hand, access to care could actually result in fewer hospitalizations, and reduced healthcare costs depending on the level of prevention concerned and the processes engaged in. Consider for example, the following. On May 26, 2006, Merck & Co. announced that U.S. regulators had approved its vaccine, Zostavax, to prevent shingles in seniors, a disease characterized by an excruciatingly painful, festering rash. Shingles results from the recrudescence of the chickenpox virus, to which about 90% of American adults have had exposure, hence are at risk of developing the disease. About 1 million cases of shingles occur in the U.S. annually, 40% to 50%, seniors. Would it not be necessary to let seniors know about this vaccine, for example via healthcare ICT-enabled targeted health information dissemination, and would such knowledge not increase access to the vaccine, which would reduce the use of the typically expensive antiviral medications, used to treat this condition, sometimes for weeks and months? Is such access to care not in the end reducing healthcare costs? Still on vaccines, a recent study has revealed a simple way to provide elderly Americans with additional protection against the yearly flu virus, giving them a higher dose of seasonal flu vaccine. The new clinical trial, which the National Institute of Allergy and Infectious Diseases (NIAID), a part of the National Institutes of Health (NIH) supported, and published in may 2006 issue of the *Archives of Internal Medicine*, suggested that a higher dose of seasonal influenza vaccine could safely, and significantly increase seniors' immune responses. This essentially protects this particularly vulnerable segment of society against influenza and its complications hence reduce influenza-associated hospitalizations, morbidities, mortalities, mostly involving seniors, thereby also reducing associated healthcare costs. Here again, is access to care not beneficial for achieving our goals of primary prevention, and by extension of secondary, and tertiary prevention regarding influenza, which affects 5% to 10% of the population yearly, and accounts for about 36,000 deaths and over 200,000 hospitalizations annually in the U.S, alone? Should other countries such as Canada, which also has a high incidence of influenza not also disseminate information regarding this vaccine to seniors and encourage them to receive it, which would increase their antibody response and confer higher protection without increasing side effects? Would appropriately deployed healthcare ICT-backed targeted health information dissemination not help achieve this goal promptly and cost-effectively? Besides the mild side effects at the injection site that the higher doses of vaccine caused in the study participants, they tolerated it well, and there were no significant differences in systemic symptoms such as fever or body aches among the participating groups. The vaccine, also approved in Europe, is not for people who have had or now have shingles, or people with weakened immune systems or HIV patients. A study showed a small increased risk of cardiovascular problems after receiving the vaccine, and some have reported side effects such as itching, and headache. Could embracing this new approach to vaccinating the elderly against influenza not help us achieve the dual objectives of delivering qualitative healthcare while reducing healthcare spending mentioned earlier? Our discussion thus far has tried to establish the significance of the disease prevention paradigm in our efforts to achieve the dual objectives mentioned above. In fact, with progress in medical research, we would soon be talking about actually pre-empting disease, which is essentially preventing genomic flaws that have the potential to result otherwise in even currently unknown diseases. There is no doubt that not having a disease in the first place is the ideal situation, and we would not even been talking about soaring healthcare costs were this, the case. However, prevention operates at other levels that offer intervention opportunities capable of not just helping us reduce healthcare costs but also providing qualitative healthcare to all. As we have argued thus far, we need to appreciate the significant role that healthcare ICT could play in our achieving these objectives. As we have also shown, it is necessary for us to conceptualize appropriately, the interplay of these technologies, the disease prevention paradigm, the dual objectives, and indeed, the prospects of attaining sustainable economic development, and fostering the survival of humankind. It is sometimes necessary to see the connection between important variables in our lives, lest we become complacent and do not take the necessary actions crucial to our survival, as the example, of recent developments regarding avian flu mentioned above shows, although we really should not wait until such a trigger before taking action. This is why we need to have a clear idea of what is at stake and the algorithm of the consequences of our actions or inactions.

With regard the importance of healthcare ICT for example, consider the following

study published in the January 30, 2006 issue of the Canadian Medical Association

Journal[6]. The authors highlighted how a benign prescribing decision could initiate

unforeseen outcomes using a case report to illustrate the point that a cascade of

unintended events could end in the development of a life threatening adverse drug

event due to the exclusion from a patient's medication list of a drug from which the

patient could have benefited used safely. Research in the acute care hospital sector[7]

indicates that computerized physician order entry (CPOE) with clinical decision

support (CDS) could improve patient safety, and prevent the scenario described

above, such improvements, especially important in long-term care, where seniors are

likely to be on multiple drug therapies, increasing the chances of errors and adverse

events, the authors noted. Long-term care facilities also often have limited access to

physician time, and few registered nurses, further heightening the chances of these

problems occurring. Having a CPOE in place would have alerted the healthcare

professionals of the bleeding risk due to interactions between the medications they

were prescribing for the patient in the case report mentioned above, for example.

Residents of long-term care facilities have relatively high rates of adverse drug events

among their residents, 9.8 per 100 resident months, over 40%, preventable[8]. Hence

the need for implementing healthcare ICT such as CPOE in these treatment settings,

and in fact, the authors noted that two such facilities, Baycrest in Toronto and the

Masonicare Facility in Connecticut, have CPOE-CDS systems in place, which should

serve as models for other long-term care settings as they implement their own

systems. CPOE systems' implementation could build on the legacy systems that some

of these facilities already have, the important thing being to ensure interoperability,

which would facilitate the integration of disparate systems such as pharmacy and

laboratory systems, and their linkage with the doctor's information systems. This

again underscores the need for us to promote the widespread diffusion of healthcare

ICT among all healthcare stakeholders. It is not only important for us to ensure

patient safety, because not doing so would not only be unethical, but could result in patients developing new health problems, some of which might be life-threatening, or their current problems becoming worse. Either way, we would be increasing morbidities and mortalities, and healthcare costs when we should be decreasing them. In other words, not ensuring patient safety would run counter to our intention to achieve the dual objectives mentioned earlier. It would also not be in keeping with the disease prevention paradigm as not only would we be creating disease, but also we would be increasing access to healthcare in a negative way, as many long-term care residents end up in hospitals due to such medical errors and the consequent adverse events alluded to in the case report mentioned above. Such hospitalizations, sometimes do not save the senior's life, and incur significant costs regardless. It is therefore, important for us to consider implementing the healthcare ICT that could help us prevent such errors. As we mentioned earlier, we should not wait for something to happen before doing so. Although some of these technologies are not cheap, for example, CPOE, their benefits over time would certainly outweigh their costs. An average 500-bed hospital with 25,000 admissions annually spent almost $8 million to implement CPOE, after paying over $1million in malpractice suit due to a medical error. Did the hospital make a wrong decision? Could the hospital be paying more in malpractice suits with error after error not implementing the technologies? What about the benefits to its patients in terms of safety, and to its image in terms of competence, hence the likelihood of more patient enrollment, and higher profitability? Do all of these not outweigh the initial and even maintenance costs of the technologies? Besides, not all CPOE run into millions of dollars to implement, costs varying with hospital size, state of legacy networks and infrastructure, the need or otherwise for wireless systems, and for integration with other hospital systems, among others. Part of the 20-hospital, seven-state Banner system, Banner Estrella Medical Center a 172-bed hospital in Phoenix, Arizona, USA, which opened 15 months ago uses a state-of-the-art electronic medical records system (EMR), with computerized physician order entry (CPOE), giving its doctors, and authorized staff instant access to patients' records. No doctor could practice at Banner Estrella without using the system, and the 400 authorized doctors use it. The training curve is intense but many nurses and physicians at every level insist that it is difficult to embrace paper charting once attuned to paperless systems. Indeed, the state governor, Janet Napolitano signed an executive order in August 2005 mandating health care providers to implement EMR by 2010, many of Arizona's hospitals now on the alert, and to speed the mandate up, the Governor formed a Health-e Connection Roadmap steering committee. Banner Estrella has hosted over a hundred groups keen to learn more about its new system, which although (the EMR and CPOE) cost it $11.5 million, many users and others agree that the benefits would eventually outweigh the cost. All the hospital's four hundred doctors could access the system in their office or home, and even write prescriptions and orders. The Arizona Republic of May 28, 2006 quoted Dr David Cohen, medical director of the hospital's ER as saying, "First of all, when I enter orders into the computer, I know they are immediately being sent to the pharmacy, lab, radiology, nursing . . . all simultaneously The second biggest gain comes from the fact that the chart is in your computer. In the paper world, if a nurse is charting on a patient's chart, I don't have the chart. That doesn't exist anymore in this system. The repository of data, and the ability to read it, is a powerful tool. " UC Davis Medical Center's EHR has also gone live according to reports in the Sacramento Business Journal of May 05, 2006. The system, which cost between $75 million to $100 million has been running at all 17 UC Davis primary-care clinics in the region since November 2005, its expansion to include direct input of doctors orders, and add hospital-based clinics and specialty programs expected over the next few years. Indeed, many other health systems in the state are in different stages of implementing EHRs. All local Kaiser Hospitals for example, have different components of EHR systems already operational. In 2007, Sutter Roseville Medical Center would be the first in Sutter to go live. Mercy's Woodland Memorial started its first phase in January 2006. More hospitals and health systems would likely follow in the state and others in the months and years ahead, and the same goes for health systems in Canada, the U.K and many other developed countries. There is no doubt that these developments augur well for our efforts to implement our disease prevention paradigm, and achieve our dual objectives of healthcare delivery mentioned earlier. It is important however, to address other issues regarding the use of these technologies, for example, the confidentiality of patient information, and the attitudinal changes that would be necessary for the end-user to embrace them. Just as important are the legislation that would pave the way for their use, and the technological sureties that would in turn facilitate the enactment of these laws. Of what use is CPOE for instance with regulations in place either barring electronic prescribing or none permitting it? These are all issues that determine access to and the quality of care, and which as we earlier mentioned are critical to conceptualize when working out the modus operandi for our disease prevention paradigm. It is also important for us to recognize the relentless forward motion of this paradigm shift, and the variety of novel healthcare-delivery concepts and modalities both emanating from and fuelling it, for examples, the concept of consumer-driven healthcare, and that of population health. The ultimate goal of the former is to nurture the well-informed and sophisticated-minded healthcare consumer able to make discerning choices on health service provision, and contributes, at least as the notion holds in the U.S, to his/her healthcare, the final common pathway of which concept would be the consumer being less indisposed, until fully healthy. This is also the ultimate goal of population health, only at a mass level. The achievement of this goal and an equally important accompanying goal for the payer, which is to reduce health spending, require the implementation of our disease prevention paradigm at all its different levels. This explains for example, a report in the May 24, 2006 issue of AP/Seattle Post-Intelligencer, that the demand for primary care providers outpaced that for specialists over the past year according to a study by Merritt, Hawkins & Associates. According to the report, requests for family doctors increased 55% from the end of March 2005 to April 1, 2006, that for internists by only 46%, during the same period. Merritt Hawkins said demand for primary care physicians is increasing with an increase in the population and its aging, yet fewer medical school graduates are entering the general medicine specialty. This is not to say that hospitals do not feature in the radar of even these new healthcare delivery models. In fact, they are crucial to certain secondary and tertiary levels health services, hence for implementing our disease prevention paradigm. The U.S, for example, would need to spend about $5 billion on its 5,000 general acute care hospitals to prepare for an avian flu pandemic observed researchers at the University of Pittsburgh Center for Biosecurity. This was according to Nancy Donegan, a spokesperson for the American Heart Association, in a written testimony to the U.S Senate Committee on Aging on May 25, 2006. After an initial $1 million spending on an average-sized 164-bed hospital, and $200,000 annually per hospital to keep it prepared, it would need an estimated $200,000 to develop a specific pandemic plan; $160,000 for staff education and training; $400,000 to stockpile minimal personal protective equipment; and $240,000 to stockpile "basic supplies". The $5 billion estimate excludes the cost of buying mechanical ventilators or of stockpiling antiviral drugs. Donegan also noted the inadequacy of current hospital capacity and staffing levels. Steven Cline, a public health official in North Carolina, agreed, observing that public health needs "a sustained and predictable stream of funding for an effective response", adding that a recent allotment of $100 million for public health departments "is far less than adequate to protect our citizens." Thus, although the federal government wants to spend $7 billion, over two to three years, for its pandemic preparation plan, none of which funds it allocates directly to hospitals, but some of which they would necessarily need.

The success of the prevention paradigm thus depends on the appropriate mix of

healthcare services in any given health system, this mix, which would in turn depend on local healthcare indicators and drivers, but which would essentially predicate on the primary, secondary, and tertiary efforts of that health jurisdiction to prevent diseases and their consequences. Underlying the success of our efforts at any of these prevention levels is the appropriate deployment of healthcare ICT in order to improve the efficiency of the processes involved in implementing its initiatives, and cost-effectively too. Thus, we need to continue to promote the widespread diffusion of these technologies, with support for one another in so doing bearing in mind the intercalations we share in not only healthcare delivery but in the survival, let alone progress of humankind. The rate of healthcare ICT adoption varies in different countries even in the developed world, the US, lagging behind by at least a dozen years other industrialized, specifically, Organization of Economic Cooperation and Development (OECD) countries in adopting healthcare ICT, in spite of spending more per capita on healthcare, according to an article in the May 2006 of *Health Affairs*. In other OECD nations, the government, health insurers, or both, pay for healthcare IT implementation, and many of them have in fact established initiatives similar to the U.S. Office of the National Coordinator for Health Information Technology to promote healthcare ICT diffusion. According to the article, Germany was the first country to commence implementing a national healthcare ICT network, billed for completion in 2006. The U.S spends the least per capita on healthcare ICT versus five other countries, total investment per capita as of 2005, 43 cents, versus, $4.93 per capita in Australia, $31.85 in Canada, $21.20 in Germany, $11.43 in Norway and $192.79 in the U.K. The report also noted the reluctance of physicians to adopt these technologies in the U.S due to concerns about loss of productivity and insufficient financial incentives, not mention costs, for example, of EHR systems, of up to $40,000 per physician in small group or solo practices. According to the researchers, "Economists recognize that use of IT in healthcare has a strong public-goods component, which means that a particular stakeholder often does not reap the full social benefits produced by new HIT investment." Indeed, many countries have started to subsidize healthcare ICT acquisition, albeit conditionally in some instances that the systems are interoperable. The U.S should consider these options and others, which might, for example, reduce the costs of these technologies, hence encourage physicians to purchase them, including the issue of testing fees for certification of healthcare ICT products. Some vendors think that the $28,000 fees are simply too high and could drive small EHR vendors out of business, and keep the prices of these technologies high. The vendors expressed these concerns at a Certification Commission for Health Information Technology (CCHIT) town hall meeting held during the Toward the Electronic Patient Record conference on May 23, 2006. The vendors were unimpressed apparently with CCHIT Chair Mark Leavitt's reminder that certification of EHRs is voluntary, claiming that they would lose market share if their products were uncertified. Furthermore, they noted the expectation by the federal government this summer to release exceptions to Stark and anti-kickback rules that would permit hospitals and others to share IT tools with physicians so long as the products meet certain standards. A few participants actually said vendors would pass certification costs to their customers, promising to raise "our prices". Leavitt on the other hand insisted that the $28,000 certification fee is less than the cost to physicians and the larger healthcare system of faulty EMR products, adding, "It's known to destroy practices (if an EMR system fails)". The Chair could not have gainsaid that considering the "mission-critical" nature of many healthcare processes and procedures. Others in the audience chided the vendors reminding them that they only need an additional sale to recoup the investment, yet others urging that matters be left to market forces to sort out. There is no doubt about the wisdom in certification, but there is a need to balance that wisdom with that of promoting the widespread implementation of these technologies, upon which condition we would likelier achieve our dual healthcare delivery objectives via implementing the prevention paradigm. Meantime, CCHIT plans to announce certified products by mid-July 2006, and physician groups among others are advising purchasers to buy only certified products. The need for support for our efforts to encourage healthcare ICT adoption is attracting attention from both the public and private sectors. Thus, two local coalitions in New York, which include local businesses, health insurers, and health systems, will utilize $4.6 million in state grants to expand the use of EHR. The groups were among the 26 regional health care networks statewide to get a piece of the $52.9 million earmarked for the state's healthcare ICT initiative that Gov. George Pataki announced May 24, 2006. Most of the funds, about $4.4 million, will go to the Rochester Regional Health Information Organization (RHIO), an extra $1.9 million raised for the RHIO project by area hospitals, insurers, and businesses, including the University of Rochester Medical Center, Eastman Kodak Co., Xerox Corp., and Excellus BlueCross BlueShield. To underscore the point about the value of healthcare

ICT in reducing healthcare costs, a feasibility study conducted before the local coalition applied for the grant indicated that RHIO would also help healthcare providers and purchasers save about $75 million yearly within six years of implementation. The savings would be for example, from rational drug prescribing and from cutting down on redundancies such as the ordering of needless tests. RHIO also plans to find additional grant money to help doctor offices, for example, purchase the hardware and software required to connect to this health information network. In fact, a project via the Greater Rochester Independent Practice Association (GRIPA), which is a partnership of physicians and hospitals in Monroe and Wayne counties, also received a grant of $227,835 through the state initiative. These developments in New York no doubt bode well for the more widespread use of healthcare ICT within the health system, and they are initiatives other states in the country and indeed, other countries, should replicate. There is no time to waste in moving our efforts to implement our disease prevention paradigm forward. We do not want to wait for catastrophe to happen before taking the action we ought to have taken to prevent it happening in the first place. Health services provision is not just a social welfare activity. It is the engine of life and of society. This fact dawns more on us as we appreciate more the essence of our increasingly integrated world. A world that requires us to revise our worldviews on healthcare delivery, and impels us to embrace such critical approaches to improving our health as implementing a disease prevention paradigm via the widespread diffusion and utilization of healthcare ICT in order to achieve our dual objectives of qualitative healthcare delivery simultaneously reducing healthcare costs.

References

1. Montgomery P; Bjornstad G; Dennis J Barnett House. Media-based behavioral treatments for behavioral problems in children. Centre for Evidence-Based Social Work, University of Oxford, Wellington Square, Oxford, UK, OX1 2ER. paul.montgomery@socres.ox.ac.uk

2. Ohinmaa1, A. Jacobs1, P, Simpson1 S, & Johnson1, J.A The Projection of Prevalence and Cost of Diabetes in Canada: 2000 to 2016. *Canadian Journal of Diabetes*. 2004; 28(2):00-00.

3. NHS acute sector expenditure for diabetes: the present, future, and excess in-patient cost of care. Currie CJ, *et al.* 1997. *Diabetic Medicine*, 14: 686-692

4. Ross, J.S., Bradley, E.H., Busch, S.H., Use of Health Care Services by Lower-Income and Higher-Income Uninsured Adults. *JAMA* vol. 295(17), 3 May 2006, p 2027̄2036

5. Woolhandler S, Campbell T, Himmelstein DU. Costs of health care administration in the United States and Canada. *N Engl J Med* 2003; 349:768-775.

6. Rochon PA, Feidl TS, Bates EW, et al. Clinical applications of a computerized system for physician order entry with clinical decision to prevent adverse drug events in long-term care. *CMAJ* 2006 Jan 3; 174(1):52-54.

7. Briggs B. CPOE: order from chaos. *Health Data Manag* 2003; 11:44-8.

8. Gurwitz JH, Field TS, Judge J, et al. The incidence of adverse drug events in two large academic long-t erm care facilities. *Am J Med* 2005; 118:251-8.

ICT and Seniors' Health

Information and communications technologies will play an increasingly crucial role

in healthcare delivery to seniors, and indeed, to all healthcare consumers in the years ahead. Considering that seniors are the most intensive users of healthcare services, and that in many countries, particularly in the developed world, we could expect more individuals to become seniors as their population ages, these technologies will therefore, be even more important for health services provision to seniors. The appreciation of the value of these technologies to healthcare delivery is not only increasing, there is also keener interest in exploiting the immense opportunities that these technologies offer. These developments are hardly surprising in view of recent developments in healthcare financing vis-à-vis the quality of healthcare delivery in many of these countries, even the developed ones. Specifically, health spending is soaring in these countries, whereas the quality of services is, some would insist, declining. This is clearly not a desirable state of affairs. On the contrary, every nation, presumably, wants to deliver qualitative healthcare to its citizens without compromising its economic well-being, and this explains in the main the increasing interests in healthcare ICT, technologies evidence shows could enable and indeed, facilitate the achievement of these dual objectives. Healthcare ICT could help improve the quality of healthcare delivery to seniors and everyone else in a variety of ways, but one that this in keeping with the direction in which healthcare seems headed is in facilitating the implementation of the disease prevention paradigm. This paradigm conceptualizes diseases on three levels of prevention, namely, primary, secondary, and tertiary prevention. Primary prevention is preventing diseases from occurring in the first place. Secondary and tertiary prevention are diagnosing and treating diseases early and promptly, and their complications, both in the short and long terms, respectively. Healthcare ICT appropriately deployed could facilitate the achievement of the objectives of any of the variety of initiatives that health systems, regardless of country, or funding model, is implementing and at any of these prevention levels. Progress in medical and technological knowledge is providing the rubric for policy formulation and the development of programs at these prevention levels. These policies and programs would require continuous reappraisal with the emergence of new knowledge further improving the quality of our health services and of healthcare delivery as healthcare ICT implementation helps deliver their goals, and assures that the future of healthcare delivery remains bright. Here then is the reason that we must not only implement these technologies but also do so on a large scale. In order words, we need to continue to promote the widespread adoption and utilization by all healthcare stakeholders of these useful technologies. With regard both, we need to put the necessary policies and mechanisms in place to encourage healthcare providers to purchase and utilize these technologies, as we would likelier reap their benefits for health service provision on a broader scale, the more widespread their diffusion and usage. The health industry seems resistive to their applications in routine patient care, although these technologies have various other uses, in facilitating the processes involved in health service provision as a whole, for examples, in the administrative and financial management domains. There are a number of reasons for this resistance, including lost productivity, costs, even technophobia. Attitudes are thawing though, albeit gradually, which is why we need to focus on change management, training, incentives to buy these technologies, and buy-in issues, among other end-user issues in our efforts to promote the widespread implementation of these technologies. Our efforts must be at once multidimensional and concerted, if we were to make any significant headway, in our quest to promote pervasive healthcare ICT deployment, and utilization in the health, and associated industries. One of the key handicaps to healthcare quality improvement is the pervasive information asymmetry that plagues the health industry, with its roots partly in the paternalistic origins of the medical profession in particular but also of the other health professions. On the other hand, many patients particularly in the developing countries where literacy levels are in general low compared to those in the developed world, also lack the skills to seek medical information, which the often limited institutional and technological infrastructure to do so, compounds. The significance of literacy in limiting knowledge of health issues for health status received research backing recently. A study researchers at the San Francisco VA Medical Center and the University of California, San Francisco conducted showed that lower literacy levels results in poor health and poor access to healthcare for seniors. The findings, published in the May 2006 issue of the Journal of the American Geriatric Society, revealed that persons aged 70 years and above with limited literacy skills are one and one half to two times as likely to have poor health, and poor health care access, versus those with adequate or higher reading ability. Seniors with limited literacy, as defined in the study, a reading level lower than ninth grade, reported poor overall health, and diabetes one and one half times, and depression, twice more, than other study participants did. One in four of the 2,512 community-dwelling seniors aged 70 to 79 years that participated in the study, which exclude those with dementia or poor physical functioning, had limited literacy, and hence might have problems reading basic health information or instructions on their medication packs and bottles. If coupled with the poor vision that diabetes causes, for example, we clearly have a major problem on our hands. Does this not call for targeted, contextualized, health information dissemination to these and other seniors and for other measures to facilitate their ability to receive, read, or listen to, and hence be able to imbibe and use health information? These are activities that healthcare ICT could enable and facilitate efficiently and cost-effectively, and are indeed, already doing so, and in which they would play an even greater role in the years ahead. The researchers also noted that individuals with a sixth-grade or lower reading level were twice as likely as the ninth-grade and above group to have poor access to health care, which not having a regular doctor or place of care, not receiving a flu shot in the past year, or lacking insurance to cover medication indicated. They also observed that seniors with a seventh- to eighth-grade reading level also had less health care access versus those that had ninth-grade literacy level, although the difference was insignificant on considering confounders. Indeed, for all results the findings held true independently of socioeconomic background and educational levels. Noted Rebecca Sudore, MD, lead author and an assistant adjunct professor of Medicine at the University of California, San Francisco (UCSF), "As a geriatrician, the results of this study break my heart…Elders already have the highest medication and disease burden. Adding

limited literacy to the list of problems makes these elders particularly vulnerable to poor outcomes, as we found in our study." There is no doubt that the findings of this study calls for urgent action to rectify this anomaly, lest we would not only be failing to deliver health services to these seniors, even the most basic not to mention qualitative, we would essentially, by our inaction, denying them access to healthcare. Here again, appropriately designed and deployed, multimedia, healthcare ICT could help these seniors, and even connect them with their healthcare providers for effective monitoring and management of their illnesses, without the need to read any health information at all. Again, as Dr. Sudore noted, "Elders with limited literacy have a hard time reading their pill bottles, managing their diseases, filling out needed forms for their care, and being able to navigate through the health care system." She added, "Unfortunately, in this study, we found that the very group of elders who would benefit from having more access to health care actually had worse access. Since the elders in our study were fairly well-functioning, problems accessing care and managing disease are likely to be even worse for frailer elders." Besides providing qualitative services to these seniors therefore, we would, by developing these specialized healthcare ICT, be contributing to our disease prevention goals, at the primary, and even secondary and tertiary levels, reducing morbidities and mortalities among these seniors, and in effect reducing health spending that we, in effect all payers, would, otherwise have incurred. This study indeed, needs replicating in other countries in order to have a clear idea of the percentage of seniors that have similar problems, which would be valuable information for policy formulation, resource allocation and program planning and execution, among other necessary activities. Besides, we need to know that the reasons why there are these links between literacy, health, and health access, a point the researchers also emphasized, possible reasons including a lack of understanding of healthcare provider instructions, the need for compliance and follow-up with treatment. There could also even be frustration with and resultant distrust of providers and health services in general, for example not being able to receive help completing insurance forms, or those needed to obtain medications. The authors noted that literacy skills are not equivalent to educational levels, hence the need for providers to communicate with and educate their patients in ways they would understand, which underscores the need for the sort of targeted, and contextualized healthcare ICT enabled, health information dissemination mentioned earlier. Indeed, Dr. Sudore advised the need for further research to determine the interventions able to prevent poor health outcomes in these prone seniors, noting the likely benefits of multidisciplinary education programs proven successful in geriatric and low-literacy populations. She also stressed that successful interventions would in the long term save money for taxpayers as "People with limited literacy skills have worse health outcomes, poor access to health care - as our study showed - and are more likely to get their care in the emergency room and to be hospitalized, which has been shown to incur higher health care costs." Should we therefore not be taking a closer look at the varieties of multimedia healthcare ICT-backed interventions that could be efficient and cost-effective in creating the enabling environment for these seniors to receive important health information? Considering that the population of many countries is aging, chances are there would be a significant number of seniors that fall into this category, regardless of their educational, and/or socioeconomic levels, hence the need for attention to ways of addressing these issues successfully. Indeed, there is increasing public awareness on the value of health information reaching the targeted audience. A recent Harris Interactive poll of 2,501 adults reported in the *Wall Street Journal Online* on May 31, 2006 found that over 80% of

U.S. adults want the results of federally funded research on health issues and other subjects to be available online gratis to doctors and the public. Eighty-one percent of respondents strongly/somewhat agreed that access to such information would help individuals living with a chronic illness or disability in "coping with that chronic illness or disability" , 62% that making research results available online free would "help speed up finding potential cures for diseases." Seventeen per cent also

strongly/somewhat agreed that scientific journals should publish the information and offer it to paid subscribers, rather than for free online. There is no doubt that such information would reach those that want it and have subscribed to it via the print media, but for those that have access to the Internet, it would doubtless reach them faster, and cheaper, even if only for the journals, key benefits underlying our call for targeted health information dissemination.

Consider a health problem common among seniors for example, constipation, a new

study that Boehringer Ingelheim sponsored, conducted on the epidemiology of which, and presented at the Digestive Disease Week congress in Los Angeles in May 20-25, 2006, offers new insights into the incidence of the problem and indicated that sufferers are simply not using the most effective treatments. The epidemiology survey explored duration and frequency of constipation in 13,879 participants from four continents. Its results indicated that 12% of people globally suffer from self-defined constipation, persons in the Americas and Asia Pacific, twice as much as Europeans, 17.3% versus 8.75%, the latter with the least rates1. The survey also showed that 25% of people suffering from constipation do not do anything to relieve their symptoms, expecting them to resolve on their own, rather than use a contact laxative, such as Dulcolax®, which is safe and effective even over the long term. Considering that not only is constipation common among seniors, but also could be sufficiently disabling to cause delirium in some case, a life-threatening condition that requires emergency medical treatment and that has a reported mortality rate of about 25%, particularly if left untreated, constipation may not be as benign as it seems. The survey showed that less than 33% of constipation sufferers that treat it use laxatives, despite research evidence that these medications are safe and effective2. Indeed, laxative use is lowest in Asia Pacific, despite high constipation rates, 17%, and despite having the highest rates of laxatives use, in the Americas, less than four in ten persons with constipation use them. According to Professor Wald, the lead author of the survey, "Sufferers continue to be highly influenced and misguided by myths surrounding constipation and it is critical to correct and overcome these mistaken beliefs. This survey reveals that on average, 40% of sufferers attempt to treat their constipation by changing their nutrition, despite extensive research showing that in fact diet and lifestyle are not necessarily to blame for the occurrence of constipation and increasing fluid and fiber intake will not definitely provide effective relief from the condition." The Professor added, "The new evidence from the survey has revealed that there is still a considerable unmet need in the treatment of constipation. It is our responsibility to make people aware of, and to offer, the best solutions for constipation, by publicizing the facts and correcting these misunderstandings." Do these observations not underline the need for targeted health information? Constipation could have many adverse consequences besides delirium in the elderly mentioned earlier, such as fecal impaction that could result in intestinal obstruction warranting surgical intervention, which some do not survive; internal, and external hemorrhoids, which could lead to enough blood loss to cause anemia, which if chronic could lead to heart failure; and many others, some potentially fatal. Should we therefore not act, as the Professor suggested? Could healthcare ICT, appropriately deployed not help in debunking these myths and changing attitudes toward this seemingly innocuous, but potentially dangerous health problem? Would we not be contributing to our efforts in achieving the dual objectives mentioned above doing so? There is no doubt that information asymmetry remains the bane of healthcare delivery, but why should we not exploit the opportunities that these technologies offer us in rectifying this perennial problem, particularly as the benefits derivable for adopting these technologies and utilizing them would far outweigh their costs, even if in the long term? A recent U.S study of

104 adults, aged 45 to 64 years, revealed that obese individuals lack awareness, that only 15% of them view themselves as obese, for example. Is this lack of awareness not an invitation to the various health problems that obesity causes or to which it has an association such as increased risk of heart disease, diabetes, high blood pressure, and arthritis? Would someone that does not see himself/herself as obese likely even focus on public health information about the consequences of obesity let alone act on it to reduce his/her weight? Unlike the 15% of participants mentioned above, 71% of individuals with normal weight and 73% of those classified as overweight, accurately assessed themselves. According to Kim Truesdale, a nutrition researcher at the University of North Carolina at Chapel Hill who presented the study at a conference in San Francisco "I think part of the disconnect is just the overall image people have when you say 'obesity.'" Is it then a denial issue, or confusion regarding Body Mass Index (BMI), which qualifies some overweight but muscle-bound individuals as having an abnormal BMI and overweight/obese, when in fact they hardly have any fat? Should we not be exploring the reasons for this lack of awareness and debunking the myths behind it? Could appropriately designed, healthcare ICT-enabled, targeted, and contextualized health information dissemination not help us in achieving this goal? Considering recent findings by the Centers for Disease Control and Prevention (CDC) that 71% of men are overweight and 31%, obese, the figures 62% and 33% for women, respectively, and experts' opinion that most Americans are not overweight due to excess muscle, and that over two-thirds of them are fat, is action on this matter not indeed urgent? The role of carbohydrates in our diet has long been controversial, and with overweight/obesity almost of epidemic proportions in many developed and in some developing countries, an important aspect of our primary prevention efforts should be letting the public know about significant research findings regarding carbohydrates and in fact any of our dietary components. Such findings include t hose of a recent study published in the May 2006 issue of the *American Journal of Clinical Nutrition* that showed that reducing carbohydrate intake could result in lowering of blood fat levels, including of cholesterol levels, even if one were not successful at losing weight. Research evidence now shows that carbohydrates, particularly simple

sugars, could lead to unhealthy fat metabolism causing fat to accumulate in the liver, as it does in the thighs and abdomen, fats that ultimately maneuver their way into the blood. Thus reducing fat deposits by reducing carbohydrate intake, would reduce fat levels in the blood, and could improve the ability of the body to break down fats in the blood. The researchers compared three groups of overweight men all of who started out on a standard diet (54% carb intake), for a week. Afterwards the researchers randomly assigned them to those that took the same, 39% and 26% carb for a three-week period. The men then ate a similar diet for another five weeks, but with their calorie intakes cut down to produce weight loss. They went through another four weeks when researchers adjusted their energy intake for weight stabilization. The findings showed that compared to the men on a standard diet, the men with the lowest carbohydrate intake showed reductions in injurious triglycerides and "bad" LDL cholesterol levels, an increase in the ratio of "good" HDL cholesterol to total cholesterol levels, and other benefits to their blood fat profile. The researchers noted these healthy outcomes regardless of the men eating or not eating, less saturated fat, and losing or not losing weight. The authors noted that the 54% carb diet is akin to the normal diet many of Americans consume by adhering to standard dietary recommendations. They recommended that individuals could reduce their carbohydrate intake to a level similar to that used in the study by simply avoiding foods such as sugary foods, white rice, pasta, white bread, which in any case are not essential to a healthy diet. They also noted the need to embark on this or any diet for that matter preferably in consultation with a dietitian to get the right balance. These findings, of course, do not, in any way suggest that it is okay to be overweight, so long as one keeps dietary carb intake low. On the contrary, the adverse consequences on health of overweight/obesity are not in doubt. There is no doubt that the public would benefit from having this information, including seniors many of who not only have weight problems that have resulted in other medical disorders such as diabetes and for whom successful changes in their carbohydrate intake would certainly help reduce morbidities and even mortalities from these medical problems. This would not only improve the quality of life (QOL) of these seniors but would also reduce their medical expenses, saving significant healthcare costs. Are these not enough reasons for us to try to deliver health information to these seniors, or should we expect them to seek it? Even if some of them seek out health information, we should not expect them to be able to keep track of even the relevant health information, considering what some would call the frenetic pace at which new medical knowledge emerges. Do these issues not speak eloquently to the need for us to embrace and act on the concept of healthcare ICT-backed targeted and contextualized health information dissemination? Health Canada and Health Canada, Eli Lilly on May 25, 2006 released an advisory that Evista, FDA approved to prevent osteoporosis and bone thinning, could increase stroke and mortality risk among some postmenopausal women living with heart conditions. Preliminary research findings of a National Cancer Institute-sponsored study released in April 2006, showed that Evista, aka raloxifene, in generic form, although not approved for breast cancer, is as effective as the breast cancer prevention drug tamoxifen in reducing breast cancer risk for postmenopausal women already prone to the cancer, and its potential for adverse events much less. A different clinical trial with over 10,000 postmenopausal women with heart conditions in 26 countries showed that 2.2 of every 1,000 women that took the medication died of a stroke, versus 1.5 per every 1,000 women taking a placebo, prompting Eli Lilly and Health Canada to recommend that women consult their physicians about the medications. This is clearly information that women ought to know about considering the increased likelihood of osteoporosis in older women, and the chances that many might be using the medication, not mention those that might be using it to prevent breast cancer. Yet, it is highly likely that many might fail to notice the information, if they did not have it delivered to them either by their doctors, or other healthcare professionals, or some way else. What would the implications be for our efforts at primary prevention were large numbers of women not to receive this information? Could this not in fact increase morbidities and mortalities among these women, with significant disease burden for them, their families, and for society? Could we not prevent such adverse implications developing ways by which we could deliver this and such important health information to women, for example, via healthcare ICT-backed, targeted, and contextualized health information dissemination?

An estimated over 20,000 Canadian women would receive the diagnosis of breast

cancer and 5,000 would likely die of it yearly, based on current estimates, according to Canada's Center for Chronic Disease Prevention and Control[3], which also noted that one in nine women in Canada would develop breast cancer during her lifetime. Breast cancer also occurs in men, although 99% of the condition occurs in women, mostly in women over 50 years old, which is why many experts recommend that women between the ages of 50 and 69 years ought to have a mammogram and clinical examination every one or two years. Despite the alarming breast cancer statistics, a recent study found gaps in knowledge of breast cancer among Ontario women, confirming what we mentioned earlier concerning how the information asymmetry that has for long compromised healthcare delivery persists even today, even in developed countries. The study, an opinion survey showed that women in Ontario have misconceptions about this major health issue regarding for examples, incidence, and risk, signs and symptoms and breast cancer screening practices. The KAP (knowledge, attitude, and Practice) survey is part of Up Front: New Perspectives on Breast Cancer, an all-inclusive inquiry into women's experience with breast cancer, which the Ontario Chapter of the Canadian Breast Cancer Foundation in collaboration with some key breast cancer stakeholders. The Institute for Social Research at York University in the survey, which RE/MAX Ontario-Atlantic Canada and the Princess Margaret Hospital Foundation Breast Centre Women's Committee funded, asked 800 Ontario women not diagnosed with breast cancer questions regarding their knowledge, attitudes, perceptions, and beliefs on breast cancer. Noted Sharon Wood, executive director, Canadian Breast Cancer Foundation - Ontario Chapter, "Significant progress has been made in raising awareness of breast cancer over the past 20 years, but the amount of information can be overwhelming to digest, and there are still some communities where information is limited". Does this not also speak to the need for targeted health information, which healthcare ICT offers us immense opportunities to conduct and efficiently and cost-effectively? The survey found that 40% of the respondents believe breast cancer is the most important health issue the contemporary woman confronts. Its findings also suggested a need to target women of non-European descent, and those in low-income groups, both the survey found less informed about breast cancer, who would less likely take part in risk reduction behaviors. Considering screening mammography alone could reduce breast cancer mortality rate by 30%, should we not in fact be more vigorous about employing multimedia healthcare ICT to disseminate relevant health information to these and other vulnerable women, for example those over 50 years, with the chances of developing breast cancer known to increase with age, and indeed, to women in general? Should it not be cause for concern that as many over 50% of the women surveyed could name only one symptom of breast cancer, lump in the breast, 11%, unable to name any, this low recognition commoner among less educated women, those with lower incomes, and those born outside Canada? Does this not call for urgent actions to assist women in identifying the signs and symptoms of breast cancer? As Wood rightly noted, "While a lump in the breast is the most commonly-known symptom of breast cancer, it is not the only one". She added, "By knowing the other signs and symptoms of breast cancer and becoming aware what is normal for them, women can be better prepared to recognize changes in their breasts that might be a sign of breast cancer." Could healthcare ICT properly deployed not help in providing women the necessary information on breast cancer? The survey even showed that many women do not know where to go to have mammograms, and x-ray breast exam that experts recommend women over 50 years have once every two years. Indeed, just 34% of the women surveyed knew the Ontario's target of 50 years for having a mammogram, 45% thought it was 40 years. Cancer Care Ontario, the agency that oversees the Ontario Breast Screening Program (OBSP), actually confirmed that just over 50% of women above 50 years receive screening. There is no doubt about the need to intensify efforts to improve awareness of breast cancer issues among women in Ontario, and in fact, worldwide, and because healthcare ICT could facilitate these efforts, it is absolutely necessary to examine ways by which we could deploy these technologies for this crucial primary prevention purposes. Still on cancer, U.K and U.S researchers recently reported details of a 10-year trial that Cancer Research UK funded and involving 1,410 women in Lancet Oncology. The researchers noted that giving 13 larger doses of radiotherapy was as effective at preventing cancer return as the standard regime of 25 small doses, findings experts believe result in simpler and more effective radiotherapy treatment, improved outcomes with less hospital visits and stays, and significant cost savings for U.K s National Health Service (NHS.) They would also no doubt improve the quality of life (QOL) of patients, save time and money spent traveling to receive treatment, and encourage better compliance with treatment, as patients currently receive radiotherapy once daily, every week day, for five weeks, and only rest at the weekend, a regime quite exhausting for many patients. Further research is under way to determine the effectiveness of this approach versus standard treatment in the long term. These findings also have important implications for resource optimization in the NHS, as there is currently a shortage of people to operate radiotherapy machines, a problem that patients requiring fewer treatments could potentially help ease. This example shows that health information dissemination could also be useful at the secondary prevention level. Would it not be easier to disseminate the information about this and other research findings to the patients that need it, which would also facilitate scheduling therapy appointments considering the limitations in the availability of professionals to handle these radiotherapy machines, thereby reducing wait times, and easing pressure of these professionals? In other words, healthcare ICT could help improve the efficiency of a variety of processes involved in healthcare delivery, some necessary spillovers from the primary implementation purpose, all working in tandem nonetheless more efficiently, to deliver care that is more effective. We could therefore, and this is often the case, be realizing expected secondary, perhaps even unanticipated gains from our investment in these technologies for an initial, specified purpose, in material, via costs savings, and human, via prompt disease diagnosis and treatment, terms. This why conceptualizing healthcare delivery in prevention terms is as heuristic as any could be. We could set out to improve certain processes and along the way not only discover new and potentially cryptic improvable processes, which might have been compromising our achievement of the dual objectives mentioned earlier, but in fact, generate new initiatives that these technologies albeit with a few upgrades here and there could also help accomplish. What's more, the processes become ongoing continuous quality improvement efforts, which would save costs, ultimately, as recent developments in the electronic submissions of health insurance claims in the U.S shows. A recent survey by America's Health Insurance Plans (AHIP) of 25 million claims that a sample of 26 health insurers processed showed that the submission of 75% of all 2006 health claims were electronically, versus 44% in 2002 and only 24% in 1995. According to the report, released in May 2006, healthcare providers submitted 30% of claims within a week in 2006, versus 19% in 2002. While there has been a reduction in lag times for provider-submitted claims, lagging submissions remain a problem, the report revealing that 29% of claims still did not come in until a month or more after the service date, 15%, more than two months or even more. The problems appears to be most prominent with paper claims, 31% of which did not reach insurers often more than 60 days after the service date, a situation that the current shift toward electronic submission would no doubt improve. Insurers are also processing claims automatically, further improving efficiency, 68% of all claims, according to the AHIP survey, 71%, and 41% of electronic and paper claims, respectively. The report also noted the cost advantages of electronic claims submission, and processing. Thus, with submissions requiring no additional information, the average processing cost for an electronic claim was 85 cents, versus $1.58 for a paper claim, pending claims that need an average of nine more processing days cost $2.05 each on the average to process. Is it any wonder that AHIP President Karen Ignani observed that "These data clearly show the best way to speed claims payment and to further reduce administrative costs is not through costly, new 'prompt pay' mandates, but rather to continue encouraging greater use of electronic claims submission." Does this not underscore the need for us to promote further the widespread diffusion of these technologies among both clinical and non-clinical healthcare stakeholders in our efforts to achieve the dual objectives of delivering qualitative healthcare cost-effectively, and efficiently? Is it not apt that the U.S Congress is enacting legislation to encourage greater use of healthcare ICT, including standardized electronic health records (EHR), with the recent 8-5 vote approval of H.R. 4157, the Health Information Technology Promotion Act, by the House Ways and Means Subcommittee on Health. To underscore the interrelatedness of these various processes, both clinical and non-clinical in making the health system work, or otherwise, could we ask if speeding up such claims not motivate providers to deliver healthcare more efficiently, and effectively, or not? A recent study published in the October 12, 2005 issue of the *Journal of the American Medical Association* assessed the effects of a pay-for-performance program in a large health plan. The study noted significant quality improvement in a physician group with a quality incentive program (QIP) for one of the three clinical measures studied, versus another without a QIP, the improvements in the other two measures, not significant. Do these findings not suggest that the widespread implementation of healthcare ICT with its prospects for process improvement, could help improve quality, and with clear expectations of incentives in place, either via speeded claims or QIPs, for examples, would this not motivate healthcare providers to invest in and implement these technologies? Incidentally, this study showed that physician groups that performed well, rather than those with most improvement received most of the bonus money in the QIPs for meeting specific targets in clinical quality scores. Indeed, many experts contend that there is a pervasive misalignment of and indeed failure to reward high quality performance in healthcare delivery in the U.S. and call for rewarding excellence adequately, and appropriately, which could no doubt improve healthcare delivery. Could not just paying for delivered services, but going a step further and rewarding the delivery of qualitative healthcare that would move us closer to achieving the dual objectives mentioned earlier, not motivate providers to implement the healthcare ICT that could enable them improve their performance, and indeed enable us to do so? The study examined quality improvements for clinical quality scores on Pap smears, mammography, and hemoglobin testing for diabetics in two groups in PacifiCare

Health Systems. The researchers compared PacifiCare's California network, which started a quality incentive program in 2003, with its Pacific Northwest group, in Oregon and Washington that did not, the former given bonuses for meeting the targets. The researchers noted that quality scores for cervical cancer screening improved 5.3% in the pay-for-performance (P4P) group, versus 1.7% in the group without (P4P,) a significant difference, but not so for the other two measures studied, mammography and hemoglobin testing for diabetics, in which both groups improved. Furthermore, the physician groups with performance above the bonus threshold before QIP implementation received 75% of the bonus payments. There is no doubt that P4P could motivate healthcare providers and improve the quality of healthcare delivery, but we must structure it properly. This could be a complex enterprise considering such issues as the involvement of multiple physicians in patient care, let us even say, for a particular disease, such as diabetes, for example, the diabetologist, nephrologist, and cardiologist, even neurologist, depending on the nature and extent of the complications of the disease. Nonetheless, one approach is as in the study above to set clear-cut quality targets based on stipulated criteria at least in the equally clear-cut cases. In other words, we need payment reforms based on a detailed evaluation of a number of clinical and other issues. In addition, we need to provide the public with the results of quality evaluation, and information on pricing, which would make the former more meaningful to the healthcare consumer in taking rational decisions regarding healthcare provider and treatment choices. This way we would be leveling the playing field, literally for consumers and providers to operate efficiently and effectively in the health market. The former would be able to patronize high quality, yet affordable providers, and providers to broaden value propositions employing sophisticated healthcare ICT and other technologies for example to improve quality at competitive prices, hence attract patronage and boost profitability, clearly, a potential win-win situation for all. There is also the need to continue to conduct studies on an ongoing basis to understand further, the various issues, for examples the regulatory, market, technological and clinical factors involved in making the execution of P4P and other payment and incentive systems succeed, or otherwise.

Some might wonder why we tie in costs so much to our discussion on qualitative

healthcare delivery. It is simply because healthcare delivery costs money, regardless of its funding system, and because money is not limitless, we cannot afford to ignore an ever-increasing health spending, as is the case in many countries today, particularly in the developed world. That, as some would argue the increasing health spending is not borne out in a corresponding increase in the quality of services delivered, compounds the problem and would no doubt jar even the most benign among us. For these reasons and many more, we need to accept the fact that the state of affairs with health services in many countries is not sustainable and we need to seek ways to rectify the problems before they assume a life of their own. Consider a *USA Today* analysis of May 25, 2005 for example, which noted that taxpayer liabilities for healthcare and sundry benefits governments promised retirees in future, increased by about $10 trillion in the past two years to $57.8 trillion or about $510,678 per household, Medicare liabilities $263,377 of the total. This is a 20% increase in taxpayer liabilities, 13% more than the inflation rate In other words, governments at various levels need these trillions of dollars to raise enough interest to meet the cost, valued in 2006 dollars, of the promised benefits. Not only must payment on this outstanding tax bill commence in due course, lest the promises made to seniors fail, but also with the costs of retirement programs billed to increase substantially as baby-boomers turn seniors in just five years time and become eligible for Medicare, in fact, for Social Security before then, in 2008. What are the implications of these figures for health spending, not to mention for future tax burden? What would happen to the country's health system if we did not start now to seek ways to achieve the dual objectives mentioned earlier, considering the expected increase in the numbers of seniors, the population segment that utilizes health services the most. Could we do something now that would in fact reduce health service utilization in future, or at least those parts of it, for example, hospitalization rates and stays, responsible in the main for driving health spending sky-high? Could investing now in the appropriate healthcare ICT help us in achieving these goals down the road? Should we not be developing innovative, healthcare ICT-enabled multimedia, and contextualized programs in the different prevention realms that would enable us achieve these dual objectives, and is it not possible to aim these programs also at address seniors' health issues? To underscore the potential impact on loss of benefits to seniors in retirement, consider the results of a survey that the Kaiser Family Foundation released on May 30, 2006. This survey, which examined the impact of the bankruptcies of two steel companies, the LTV Corporation and Bethlehem Steel, on health coverage for the firms' retirees and dependents, noted that it left about 200,000 of them without retiree health coverage in 2002 and 2003. The report also offers a hint into the effect of a tax credit that Congress passed in 2002 aimed at providing provisional support to workers and retirees in "distressed" industries. It found that notwithstanding, almost 75% of respondents had received replacement coverage or a supplement to their Medicare coverage many insisted the loss of benefits significantly disrupted their retirement. Twenty six percent of the 55 to 64 year old respondents said that they use the 2002 Trade Adjustment Act's health insurance tax credit, which funds up to 65% of health insurance costs for eligibles, who also receive refunds from the IRS if they owed less tax than the credit amount. The loss of health coverage meant that for about 50% of retirees 65 years or under, he/she or a spouse had to delay retirement or return to employment, about 25% digging deep into their savings or assets to fund their healthcare costs or premiums. Those uninsured were twice as much likely to go without or postpone needed healthcare on costs grounds. The survey also found that Medicare provided primary coverage for retirees and spouses aged 65 years and above. Medicare HMO or supplemental coverage covers 74% of respondents. However, 51% of all Medicare-eligible respondents without supplemental coverage said that they "often" or "sometimes" were not compliant with prescribed medications due to cost, versus 29% with a supplemental coverage. There is no doubt about the need for seniors not only to have access to care, but not to lack care because of costs. Besides the underlying ethico-moral issues involved in such lack of access to care, and the burden of illness on the seniors and their families, seniors would be less healthy and end up in the ER, perhaps hospitalized, which would in the end cost more to the taxpayer than did they not lack access to healthcare in the first place. The need for seniors to have access to healthcare and the possible consequences of this access lacking as the above scenario shows, also applies to other countries besides the U.S. These examples not only illustrate the need for seniors to have access to care on the one hand, but also not to promote excessive use of hospital services in particular on the other. They also highlight the need for us to design and implement effective services, enabled by healthcare ICT, to deliver health services to seniors at the different levels of the disease prevention paradigm. An example of such efforts is the recent design by the U.S National Institute on Aging (NIA) a part of the National Institute of Health of two easy-to-read booklets on Alzheimer's disease (AD) and memory loss, in which it replaced medical and technical language with plain language, stories, photographs, and other features to facilitate readers' understand of their content. This is the sort of targeted health information that we advocate, in paper form, although these efforts could also be in electronic, documentary-type multimedia formats, for example, which might work better for certain elderly populations. According to Richard J. Hodes, M.D., the NIA director, "Our goal was to produce strong, clear materials to make information about AD and memory loss accessible to everyone, including those with limited literacy skills." He added, "These booklets also are excellent starting points for anyone who needs basic information about AD and memory problems, regardless of reading capability." The NIA produced the booklets after local field-testing, and interviews with care givers and further testing for overall appeal, format, graphic elements, comprehension, cultural appropriateness, and "self-efficacy", which latter measures the individual's appreciation of the significance of acting on emergent signs of AD or serious memory loss, and the incorporation of feedbacks from these and various other sources. As previously noted, part of our efforts to implement disease prevention services involves information dissemination to healthcare providers as well as patients themselves, as the following example regarding stroke shows. German scientists, who presented their findings to the recent European Stroke Congress in Brussels, reported that a rare genetic disorder is the cause of some strokes in young people. The researchers found that 4% of more than 700 stroke patients aged 18 to 55 years also had Fabry disease, strokes occurring ten years earlier in persons with this disease. Although the findings apply to a small number of individuals, it nonetheless revealed a preventable and treatable cause of stroke, Fabry disease, caused by a missing or faulty enzyme that the body requires to process oils, waxes, and fatty acids, which then accumulate to dangerous levels in the eyes, kidneys, nervous system, and cardiovascular system. Persons with the disease could die early due to renal, cardiac, or cerebrovascular complications, which enzyme replacement therapy could slow and prevent, which is why all doctors and healthcare professionals, at least those that treat stroke need to be aware of this disease. Unlike for men and women that do not have Fabry disease for who the average age for having stroke is 48 years, it is 38 and 40 years, for men and women, respectively with the disease. This research underscores the need for screening for Fabry disease in young people. It also suggests that we need to consider it a probable cause of a cryptogenic stroke in young persons, an important aspect of implementing our disease prevention paradigm, which could reduce the burden of stroke and its complications down the road. Healthcare practitioners in particular should be prime movers in the health-information dissemination efforts to facilitate the screening process, and it would, no doubt be more efficient for them to do so having the appropriate healthcare ICT implemented. We should not only encourage them to implement these technologies, they also need to embrace and use the technologies. In the UK, a recent BBC News survey showed that doctors want a review into the £6.2bn NHS computer project, the ICT upgrade intended to connect 30,000 GPs to nearly 300 hospitals in a major revamping of the NHS ICT network. One important part of this upgrade is the choose and book, which is a system t hat enables patients to book hospital appointments at a place, date, and time convenient to them from GP surgeries, almost 10m such referrals made annually. Another is the NHS care records service, which is an electronic database of patient medical records for 50 million patients that would give NHS staff nationwide, access to patient information at the point of care (POC). The upgrade also includes capabilities for electronic prescriptions. With over 325m prescriptions made annually, an electronic version would replace the current paper-based system by 2007. This would enable patients to pick up repeat prescriptions from any pharmacy nationwide. However, the survey, which 447 hospital doctors and 340 GPs completed, showed that 50% of the GPs thought that the "choose and book" online booking system was poor/fairly poor. This could be a major setback for the project if nothing happened to understand and rectify the problems the doctors had with the system, other parts of which Ministers incidentally concurred were behind schedule, hence guzzling more than their budgets, the EHR, for example, lagging over two years behind schedule. According to the NHS, the "choose and book system", which it has been promoting, has helped make 400,000 appointments so far, which would no doubt help reduce wait times, and improve accessibility to healthcare. These would in turn reduce morbidities and mortalities, and healthcare costs, which are cogent reasons that it is necessary to address the problems that doctors have with the system urgently. This is more so considering that, as many as four out of five GPs, as the results of the BBC Radio 4's File on Four survey show, had access to the computer system, but 50% said that they hardly or never use it, with only about 20% acknowledging that the system was good/fairly good. Indeed, 85% of the doctors urged an independent expert technical review of the whole scheme to ensure its fundamental viability. Interestingly, when asked if the cost of the upgrade was a good use of NHS resources, almost two-thirds of GPs and hospital doctors did not think so, which is a clear indication of the urgent need to tackle the issue of acceptance of healthcare ICT in the U.K. This issue is not peculiar to the country but pervasive among healthcare professionals in many others, developed and developing. The reasons for this seeming antipathy toward healthcare ICT in the medical professional are legion, but one of the most often mentioned in researches is lost productivity. This however, underscores the need for improvement in the technologies but also the need for training and the learning curve for some of these technologies, particularly for many doctors that are not tech-savvy could indeed be steep, not to mention the costs in time, regardless of prior knowledge or interest in healthcare ICT. Privacy and confidentiality issues also concern many doctors, as do logistics problems for example involved with booking hospital appointments from GPs' surgeries. There is no doubt that there are problems along the road to widespread healthcare ICT implementation, and that of end-user buy is perhaps as crucial, if not more than implementing the technologies themselves. The delay in implementing EHR in the U.K could mean that electronic records might not be deployable in the country until early 2008, which creates immense opportunities to mobilize the appropriate agencies to embark on massive change management exercises for the healthcare professionals. As with any new enterprise, there would also be teething problems, some anticipated, others, not. Solutions to some of these problems would come easy, others would be essentially intractable, at least in the immediate, possible even in the short term. Nonetheless, we must keep seeking these solutions and moving the enterprise forward, knowing the prospects are real of being able to achieve our dual objectives of qualitative healthcare delivery while simultaneously reducing costs. Reports indicate that software development is one major cause of delay with some of these technologies, for example the EHR in the U.K upgrade project. This is hardly surprising considering the vary nature of software, with millions of codes sometimes required to write and execute for just one product, and sometimes even just an aspect of it, among other inherent problems. There are again, many technical issues involved that could cause such a delay for examples, those regarding verification and validation, or hopefully not, even flawed requirements analysis. Thus, software developers and vendors need to be active partners in our efforts to achieve the dual healthcare delivery goals, as they are major stakeholders in these efforts. Considering that healthcare delivery often involves matters of life and death, there is no room for errors and software must be very near if not perfect. Here we begin to see the interrelationships of various factors in our ability to achieve the dual objectives. This underscores the need for a more widespread campaign to promote the pervasive diffusion of healthcare ICT, not just in the health but also in related industries, for example, the insurance industry. It is also important to promote the use of these technologies in the financial, administrative, and other domains that operate in tandem to ensure the delivery of cost-effective, yet qualitative health services.

With regard the variety of interlocking issues that challenge us in our efforts to achieve the dual goals, let us examine the problems with healthcare ICT implementation in the UK mentioned above a little further. The fact is, there is not much time to waste in implementing these technologies for a number of reasons including for example the state of affairs with pensions in the country, and its possible impact on future health services provision. By 2020, an estimated 26% of the UK population will be over 60 years of age; by 2050, 38%. Millions lack an occupational pension, and many more workers will have to rely solely on the state post-retirement, which would worsen with employers shutting off munificent final salary pension schemes, which helped reduce reliance on the state, and which led to so much frustration, even strike actions, in the early 2000s. The Adair Turner-headed Pensions Commission in 2004 highlighted the shortfalls in the country's retirement provision, with an estimated 11.3 million workers not making any pension contributions. Of those who were, many, pittance. About 12 million persons aged 25 years and over, for example, saved next to nothing, experts noting then that without increasing taxes or retirement ages, pensioners will suffer a 30% decline in relative incomes, borne out by recent events for examples, the planned increase incrementally to 68 years by 2044, and the restoration of the state pension and earnings link. The link would be by 2012, the latest, concerns about this not materializing because of a dispute on its details including funding between the Prime Minister and the Chancellor, now laid to rest with a recent deal announced between them. In addition, in response to the report of the Pensions Commission Government also wants to establish a new savings scheme with automatic enrolment for staff and compulsory employers' contributions. The aging population is at the core of these pensions-problems, with increasing fewer taxpayers of working age to pay everyone's pensions, a demographic zero-sum game slamming pensions everywhere, public and private, the stock market not particularly endearing enough and corporate scandals discouraging enough to boost people s interest in pension schemes. Higher taxes, increased savings, and retirement age are options to tacking these problems but are politically dicey. These issues might have profound impact on the resources available for health spending in the U.K in the near future, or at least make it difficult for it to continue to soar relentlessly as it does currently. These issues underscore the need for urgent steps to curtail health spending while not compromising the quality of healthcare delivery, both that the widespread implementation and utilization of healthcare ICT promises, and could deliver. Within a decade, about 50% of the UK adult population will be aged over 50, yet a recent research conducted for Heyday, a new group in the U.K, to address concerns regarding persons born between 1946 and 1965, shows that 41% of individuals in their 50s have not started actively planning for retirement. Furthermore, even if, as this survey by Heyday, set up by Age Concern, and similar to the American Association of Retired Persons (AARP), of 1,770 persons shows, 48% of these baby-boomers want to work well past the current retirement age of 65 years, ageism stands in their way, as 64% gracefully acknowledged. This is besides the vagaries of the prevailing economic climate, with employers, ever ready to slice the labor force in the event of a downturn in economic growth. In all, the need for sustainability in the U.K health system calls for the necessary steps to achieve the dual objectives mentioned earlier in our discussion. The call in fact applies to all health systems regardless of whether publicly or privately funded. There is no doubt about the role a country s funding structure of its health system in issues such as universality and accessibility, among others, issues germane to the quality of healthcare delivery in the long term, and which healthcare ICT appropriately deployed could help improve the health system s funding structure regardless. These issues also partly explain the differential scorecards the health systems in Canada, the U.K, and the U.S, received recently based on new research findings. According to a recent study published in the May 03, 2006 issue of the Journal of the American Medical Association, white, middle-aged Americans, even the rich, are much less healthy than their English counterparts, the former having higher rates of diabetes, heart disease, strokes, lung disease and cancer, the findings true regardless of income or education level. Yet, the U.S. health care spending is twice, $5,200 per person that of England per citizen in adjusted dollars, the study supporting previously established findings that the U.S. spends more on health care than any other industrialized country, but lags behind in rankings of life expectancy. Too little exercise, excessive stress, the U.S obesity epidemic, and a variety of reasons proffered have not diminished interests in finding explanations for these observations. The researchers, who studied people, aged 55 to 64 years, the average age of the samples the same, even included non-Hispanic whites in the study to eliminate the effect of racial differences. The study found that high-income persons in both countries were healthier than middle-and low-income persons were, but the health status of high-income Americans was similar to that of the low-income English, compounding the mystery. The relative poor showing of the health status of Americans is well known, and according to the World Health Organization (WHO), Americans rank behind not less than twenty other nationals in this regard, but the findings of this study are new and add even newer dimensions to the matter. Could the findings be due to more ethnic-diversity, some ask, given that the health of minorities for a variety of reasons is in general worse than that of whites? However, as noted earlier, the researchers adjusted for this potential ethnic bias. Previous studies have contrasted the U.S. with other countries regarding availability of and access to healthcare services, healthcare expenditures, service utilization, and other parameters, but this is the first to address the prevalence of chronic conditions, incidentally, more prevalent among seniors, and considering the age groups studied, prevalence we should expect they might carry forward into the senior years. Could physical activity be the reason as one of the researchers suggested, although not likely the only one? Some even mentioned financial insecurity, household income increase unknown in all but the top fifth of Americans since the mid-1970s, that of the English improving on the contrary. Were this in fact the case, are the advantages of the English sustainable in the long term considering the pensions crisis mentioned earlier, and in particularly with the necessary measures not taken to reduce spiraling healthcare spending? Does this not speak to the need to eschew delaying the adoption of healthcare ICT that could help reduce healthcare spending while in fact improving the quality of healthcare delivery to the bargain? In a similar vein, would the health status of Americans not improve addressing the process issues that bog down the country's health systems, both clinical and non-clinical, which are the real reasons for its seemingly unwieldy healthcare delivery systems? It is unlikely that the stress of striving for the American dream has more damaging effect on health than that of striving for the English, barring any significant genetic differences in the stress reactions, and considering that, both countries have a social welfare system. Besides, even if the safety net of the U.S were flawed, does it explain why those that have achieved the American dream could only be as healthy as those that presumably have yet to achieve the English dream? Furthermore, does the National Health Service (NHS) in particular considering its many administrative, clinical, including wait times, and financial problems, explain the better health of the high-income English, even if it did that of the low-income? Even if it did, does it explain why Americans with insurance were in such relatively poor health? There is no doubt about the heuristics of exploring the differences in health status revealed in this study utilizing the disease prevention paradigm. We would then be able to see vividly, the natural histories of these chronic health problems and the differences in the processes involved in their evolution, between the two countries, after all, it is not that they exist in one or the other country. This revelation would enable us see all the processes, both clinical and non-clinical, including their determinants and outcomes, the processes and variables constituting the foundation upon which we would formulate the necessary policies within the context of our strategic objectives, that would determine the required healthcare ICT-enabled initiatives we would act on in a change continuum of healthcare quality improvement. Another recent study billed for publication in the July 2006 issue of the *American Journal of Public Health,* compared the health of Canadians and Americans. The study found that Canadians are healthier, have better access to healthcare, yet spend half of what Americans spend on their health system, $6,000 for every American. They also found that Canadians were 7% likelier to have a regular doctor, 19% less likely to have their health needs go unmet than Americans, who were more than twice as likely to give up go without needed medicines due to cost. With income, age, sex, race and immigrant status taking into consideration, the differences became even more prominent, with Canadians 33% likelier to have a regular doctor and 27% unlikelier to have an unmet health need. The study also showed that Americans had higher rates of almost all serious chronic disease, for examples obesity, diabetes and chronic lung disease, although they smoked cigarettes less. This study's researchers suggest the biggest obstacle to health care in the U.S is cost, responsible for more than seven times more U.S. residents forfeiting needed healthcare compared to Canadians, the uninsured particularly vulnerable, with 30.4% having an unmet health need due to cost. Costs also explain why low income and minority patients fare better in Canada, but could inefficient processes be responsible for the high costs of care in the U.S or not? Considering that unlike U.S/U.K study, insured Americans and Canadians had about the same rates of disease, and that uninsured Americans worsened the overall figures, does it only have to do with the benefits of access to healthcare? If so, why does this not explain the differences between the health status of the Americans and the English, as noted above? There is no doubt that access to care is crucial and must have a hand these differences, at least on the aggregate, after all the more persons that lack access to care the less health the population would be overall. Yet, even then, it would unlikely explain all the observed differences and it would be in the end a matter of understanding the intricacies of the underlying processes involved largely, with healthcare delivery in either health system. Thus, could the appropriate deployment of healthcare ICT not improve these processes hence improve healthcare delivery and reduce healthcare costs? Would reducing healthcare costs without compromising the quality of healthcare delivery not become possible with the widespread implementation of healthcare ICT, as we have discussed so far? By improving the quality of healthcare delivery, would healthcare ICT not be contributing to making people healthier, and with improved health, would service utilization, in particular hospitalization rates and stays not be less, thus further reducing health spending? Would this not free up scarce resources that could go into other important social programs such as education, or any other for that matter, for example seniors pensions and other benefits as discussed earlier? The study also found that Canadians wait, on average, three times more than Americans for medical t reatment, which suggests that the country's health system also needs to examine its processes and implement measures to improve them, here again, which appropriately deployed healthcare ICT could help achieve, and cost-effectively too. The point here is that no matter the funding structure of a health system, healthcare delivery is a conglomeration of intricately intertwined processes, which we need to understand in detail for us to determine its flaws and rectify them using the right healthcare ICT, and other suitable solutions. This underscores the need for cautious interpretation of such findings as mentioned above, particularly in order to avoid complacency of the parts of the systems that fared better, and more particularly to appreciate the contextual nature of process evaluation, hence of the applicable quality improvement strategies. Thus, for example, the issue of wait times remains sticky in both Canada and the U.K, and these studies would unlikely change the views of the citizens of these two countries regarding the need to fix these problems. Indeed, in the case of Canada, it has resulted in a landmark Supreme Court ruling in *Chaoulli v. Quebec,* which has rekindled a long-standing debate on the continuing status of the country's cherished Medicare, the publicly funded health system, with some calling for a parallel private health system. In the U.K, it is equally topical, and partly responsible for the various initiatives that have increasingly infused private funding arrangements into the country's publicly funded health system. As we have argued thus far, every health system needs its processes revisited on an ongoing basis, in light of developments such as the "wait times" issues, and even such studies as mentioned above, although it should routinely, periodically, as part of an internal audit effort to ensure continuous quality improvement. Canada and the U.K for examples might be spending less money to obtain better health outcomes than the U.S does but could these latter countries obtain even better outcomes for even lesser health spending, or put differently, could they afford an ever-increasing health expenditure or could they curtail these soaring expenditures yet in fact improve the quality of healthcare delivery? The answer is a resounding yes, provided of course they are willing to decompose and understand the processes involved in the healthcare delivery processes, which by the way are not static, as medical knowledge and disease emergence, patterns and prevalence continually evolve, and embark on a healthcare ICT-based continuous quality improvement efforts. This holds true for any health system in the world. The results of a study published in the May issue of the *Annals of Internal Medicine* are instructive. According to this study, primary care doctors who work in areas with the most medical resources, for examples, hospital beds, laboratory services, and specialists, reported being less satisfied with the quality of care they provide than those working in areas that have less resources did, Medicare spending 58% higher in the former areas. Researchers at Dartmouth Medical School interviewed 6,000 physicians who treat Medicare patients nationwide, and found that 50% of doctors in high-intensity healthcare areas said that they could obtain elective hospital admissions for their patients, versus 64% in low-intensity areas. Doctors in the former were less likely to say that they obtained adequate hospital stays, strong specialist referrals, or high-quality diagnostic imaging services, for patients, and were less likely to say that they were satisfied with their careers. The researchers noted that the increased demand for resources in high-intensity health care areas creates an endless demand-supply cycle, which perhaps explains the dissatisfaction of the doctors in the midst of plenty, literally. Does this not speak to the need to pay attention to processes? Could this not be part-explanation for some of the observations made in the comparative studies mentioned earlier? Does this study not also imply that the increasing health spending does not guarantee service quality? Could we assert that these unhappy doctors would offer the highest quality healthcare? Could we not improve the productivity of these doctors by improving the processes involved in their healthcare delivery activities? According to Lawrence Casalino, professor of health studies at the University of Chicago, "The implications (of the study) are important; it's not that we need to pour more money into the system, and it's not that we need more hospital beds and more specialists." In fact, earlier studies conducted in Dartmouth had noted that costlier health care and more services do not improve patient outcomes, and researchers have estimated that 30% of Medicare expenditure is on needless care. Is the U.S Tort system in fact not also fuelling costs nurturing the "defensive Medicine" that results in a lot of the needless care? Are these not some of the reasons health spending in the U.S, and possibly elsewhere is skyrocketing, and could we not prevent this? Could we not make health systems work better via healthcare ICT implementation and utilization? The fact is, we could, and we not only want health systems to work, but to work better all the time. This is the only way some "disruptive disease" such as HIV/AIDS or avian flue would not catch us flat-footed, literally. Countries could also learn form one another regarding measures implemented that seem to be proving effective in not only preventing diseases but also regarding even other non-clinical aspects of the healthcare delivery processes. However, as noted above, the recipient must apply these measures to its health system contextually, which is why the U.K, although introducing private funding arrangements into an essentially publicly funded health system, is not importing the American style of private health system or that of any other country for that matter wholesale.

Efforts to promote the widespread diffusion of healthcare ICT into health systems

must continue apace. As noted earlier, changes are occurring in various domains such as demographics, medical knowledge base, and regarding technological innovation that we cannot afford to rest assured that our health systems, in whatever country, is working and needs no improvement. Whereas in fact, health spending is increasing, some would say exponentially in many countries, particularly in the developed world, yet resources are limited, if not in fact dwindling. These combinations call for urgent action to achieve the dual objectives of qualitative healthcare delivery simultaneously reducing health spending. Efforts are indeed afoot in many countries to implement healthcare ICT on a large scale within the health systems, particularly in the developed countries. However, we need to address other important issues besides investing in these technologies, for example, encouraging the end-users, particularly healthcare providers, to embrace, invest in, implement, and utilize these technologies. There is no doubt that there is currently some resistance among these professionals to healthcare ICT implementation and use. The reasons for this resistance are many, cost also being a major one. However, and despite the cost issues that no doubt make it difficult for many providers in small and solo practices to be able to purchase EHR systems, the consensus amongst experts is that these technologies could improve the efficiency and quality of healthcare delivery. Indeed, a recent Commonwealth Fund-supported research to examine the costs and benefits of these technologies, in particular for solo or small group practices, where almost 80% of U.S. doctors operate found the average start-up costs for small group practices with EHRs, were $44,000 per physician, or nurse practitioner, average ongoing costs, $8,400 per physician per annum. As high as they may seem, the researchers also found that the average practice would recoup these costs in less than three years and, after that, profit substantially. The financial benefits averaged $33,000 per physician per annum, savings from two main sources, namely increased coding levels resulting in improved billing, and increased efficiency from reduction in personnel costs, with every practice reporting some savings, ranging from $1,000 to $42,500 per physician, or nurse practitioner per annum. Other benefits such as legibility, better data organization, and easy accessibility to patient records even from home, also improved efficiency. The study[4], published in the Sept/Oct. 2005 issue of *Health Affairs,* Sept./Oct. 2005, also observed that many of the doctors worked longer hours initially, and some confronted significant financial risks, such as long payback periods, billing difficulties, loss of data, problems that with time, they typically overcame. The researchers recommend the formulation of policies to provide incentives and support services to assist practices improve the quality of their care by using EHRs. This study clearly supports our assertion thus far of the benefits of healthcare ICT in improving the quality of healthcare delivery, cost-effectively, with all involved deriving some benefits, clinical and/or pecuniary from these technologies, even if in the long term. Indeed, all the practices involved in this study conducted at least some quality improvement (QI) related EHR activities, although just two of them used the EHR systems rigorously to systematically improve chronic and preventive care, and some did not in fact exploit the technologies to the fullest, for example, using practice-set reminders or generating reports on provider performance. We should not only encourage healthcare providers to purchase, implement, and use healthcare ICT, emphasizing the numerous benefits of these technologies as the findings in this study showed, we should also encourage the use of these technologies for specific quality improvement efforts, offer incentives for such efforts, and compensate those that do so appropriately. Without such incentives and recompense, deliverable via such payment systems as P4P for example, it would likely be difficult to get providers to commit the time and efforts to learning the use of the many features of the EHR, for example, for quality improvement purposes. We might also minimize costs, time and monetary, to providers offering financial and other support for implementation-related activities such as office do-over, to encourage quality improvement use of the technologies, particularly as EHR software training and installation costs alone on the average were $22,038 per physician, or nurse practitioner, software constituting about one-third of overall costs, according to this study. The U.S Agency for Healthcare Research Quality (AHRQ) has developed a guide, "Pay for Performance: A Decision Guide for Purchasers," released in April 2006 that examines the decisions public and private purchasers of health care services need to make when designing and implementing P4P programs. The guide has 20 questions in four phases, namely, contemplation, design, implementation, and evaluation, and each question reviews the possible options, potential effects, and consequences. It also provides evidence from empirical evaluations and economic theory to help purchasers make informed decisions on P4P implementation, which could be complex under certain circumstances as mentioned earlier. Such guides would not only facilitate the implementation efforts, but would make the benefits realizable from a P4P more likely achievable, with the quality improvements in healthcare delivery thus engendered helping to move us closer to realizing the dual objectives mentioned earlier. AHRQ developed the guide for public and private healthcare services purchasers, including health plans planning to sponsor a P4P initiative, which AHRQ broadly defined as any type of performance-based provider payment arrangements, including those that target performance on cost measures. There is no doubt that it would serve its intended purposes remarkably, and with consumer-directed health plans gaining increasing currency, according to the a recent study, it would be an invaluable quality improvement tool that would further promote the wider acceptance of consumer-driven healthcare delivery model. The U.S. Government Accountability Office (GAO) report released on May 30, 2006, noted that the number of U.S. residents that enrolled in consumer-directed health plans increased from about three million in January 2005 to about six million by January 2006, the policies typically combined with health savings accounts (HSA). They must also have a minimum deductible of $1,050 for a single person and $2,100 for a family. According to the GAO report, the number of employers offering high-deductible insurance plans to workers rose from 1% in 2004 to roughly 4% in 2005, about 30% of enrollees, previously uninsured. As the consumer-driven healthcare model becomes more widely accepted, the need for the healthcare consumer to have the right information at the right time to take the necessary decisions regarding their health in a rational manner becomes even more urgent. The high-deductible plans have critics no doubt, some for example claiming that it best suits younger, healthier workers, others that employers use it as a ploy to shift costs to employees. Nonetheless, we cannot ignore the facts that not only are many more enrolling in these plans, but also that in the process they are reducing the numbers of the uninsured. The more Americans gain access to healthcare, the healthier the populace would be, as this increasingly discerning population of healthcare consumers demands qualitative healthcare, which would impel healthcare providers to embrace and nurture quality including investing in the means by which to achieve this quality, for example in healthcare ICT, in order to remain competitive. Prices would also fall as competition heats up, making health services even more affordable, and many more Americans able to access health services. It is easy to see how ICT would trigger and sustain a healthcare quality cycle that would enable us achieve the dual objectives mentioned earlier. In fact, there is increasing research evidence that these technologies do indeed, improve healthcare quality as the following study shows. In May 2006, Mathematica Policy Research, Inc., released the results of a study it carried out for the Centers for Medicare & Medicaid Services via the Delmarva Foundation. The aim of the study was to determine if the use of six specific types of information technology had improved quality of care. The survey involved 650 senior hospital executives asked questions to determine the benefits of EHR capabilities such as e-prescribing and electronic lab orders at their hospitals. The most important benefits of healthcare ICT that respondents reported were more timely clinical information, diagnosis, and treatment, next to which were reduced medical errors and improved patient safety. The researchers concluded that many of the hospital executives felt that healthcare ICT had advanced the quality of care in several important ways, with most hospitals acknowledging improved quality due to the healthcare ICT initiatives that they started. There is though, an urgent need for the establishment of timeliness measures including of health information availability and accessibility, particularly at the point of care (POC), and of diagnosis and treatment, all of which would improve documentation of the benefits derived from implementing these technologies. The need for widespread healthcare ICT implementation in order to obtain more accurate comparative data on quality-related healthcare ICT issues, particularly between different healthcare settings, for example between those accredited by Joint Commission on Accreditation of Healthcare Organizations (JCAHO) and those not and for different health conditions in these settings is pressing. This would enable a deeper understanding of the operational processes that would help us achieve higher quality improvement. The study highlighted the need for healthcare ICT to be efficient in data extraction for quality reporting, and the fact that electronic reminders and prescribing lagged behind other types of healthcare ICT, a situation that needs urgent rectifying considering the values of these features in reducing medical error rates and improving patient safety. There are though, technical implementation hassles one should acknowledge regarding the said features that might be the reason for the lag. However, they are certainly not the only problem, considering that many health jurisdictions do not have the required legislation to enable the use of e-prescribing for example, for reasons such as privacy and confidentiality and problematic certification issues. There would indeed be many issues to deal with right away given this increasing interest in consumer-driven health plans for the scenario described above to materialize, which is to intensify our efforts to promote the widespread diffusion of healthcare ICT. Some would even advocate offering healthcare providers some incentives to adopt these technologies in order to speed this process up. Healthcare ICT no doubt costs money; an estimated $400 billion over five years to build a national health information network (NHIN) for example, according to a study published in the August 02, 2005 issue of the *Annals of Internal Medicine*. The research team led by Rainu Kaushal, M.D., M.P.H., of Brigham and Women's Hospital in Boston, evaluated the status of healthcare ICT within the health system, and projected the costs of a model NHIN, which would have electronic health records (EHRs), secure electronic communication between patients and providers, and electronic claims submissions and eligibility verification capabilitiess. It would also enable the end-user to view and share test results, and would have computerized physician order entry (CPOE), and electronic prescribing features. Despite the huge costs of such a network, the researchers also noted that the savings that hospitals, physicians, and insurers would derive from improved operational efficiencies could considerably offset, and indeed recoup, the expense. The study observed that a network connecting U.S. health care providers to insurers, pharmacies, home health agencies, and clinical laboratories would cost $156 billion in capital investment over five years and $48 billion in annual operating costs. With capital expenses and operating costs combined, the total cost of a network with the ideal features mentioned earlier would be about $400 billion over five years. This stunningly expensive project would however, by improving communication between physicians, hospitals, pharmacies, labs, and insurers would reduce unnecessary testing, administrative and labor costs, resulting in overall savings to the tune of $77.8 billion annually, according to another study published in the January 9, 2005 issue of *Health Affairs*6. What we need to continue to do is to present facts such as these to hospital executives, physician groups, and insurers so that they see the value of investing in these technologies, and be rest assured that they could recoup their investments over time. Admittedly, we have not succeeded greatly in so doing thus far, considering the painfully slow pace of healthcare ICT adoption in certain segments of the health industry. Nonetheless, this is essentially work in progress, considering that we have cogent reasons some of which we have discussed in this paper to work fervently toward achieving the dual healthcare delivery objectives mentioned earlier. Experience in the U.S for example indicates that besides some of the country's largest hospital systems, the response to coming up with the initial financial outlay in the healthcare ICT required for the NHIN, has been at best lukewarm, which is why some advocate offering incentives to healthcare providers to invest in these technologies. Considering the potential problems health systems face around the world and in particular in developed countries in view of the anticipated spike in the numbers of seniors in just a few years ahead, this delay in embracing the technologies that could help cushion the adverse effects of these demographic, and other changes, is unmistakably troubling, and could prove exceedingly costly. Many experts do not feel that government should foot the bill in the U.S, but this would likely be the case in countries such as Canada, and the U.K., to a large extent, individual healthcare providers that are self-employed funding their own technologies, albeit perhaps with provincial or other assistance and incentives as is the case in Alberta, for example. In the US, some experts feel that the influence of governments would even be more profound regarding our bid to promote the widespread diffusion of these technologies if they purchased healthcare services from health care providers that have implemented and are using healthcare ICT. There is no doubt that even in the U.S and as is already happening, governments have a critical role to play in funding the fundamental technical infrastructure of such a network, besides their roles in offering incentives to providers to implement these technologies, for example increased recompense via Medicare for healthcare providers that have implemented healthcare ICT. Further, there ought to be even more incentives for those providers that are utilizing these technologies in innovative ways to foster our chances of achieving our disease prevention goals. There is no doubt that providers, health plans and hospitals should have a financial stake in the technologies in their practices. This would ensure that they use them for the purposes for which bought, besides the desire to recoup their investments, not only via broadening their value propositions to their clientele, but also as adherence to quality could attract incentives and rewards as mentioned earlier. Issues such as convincing providers to come up with the initial investment remain potential problems. Further, some might see these technologies as anything but a blessing down the road as improvement in health status might mean less patronage, not to mention the form and standards for a NHIN might change with possible loss of investments, and the price wars that they could trigger in order to remain competitive might make some practices moribund. These are concerns that we also need to address, in order to reassure these providers, and get them to invest in the technologies, and we might actually also have to offer financial incentives along the way, in addition to providing further evidence of the clinical and financial benefits of these technologies in the long term. It would certainly be likely necessary to prop up smaller, rural, and solo practices by offering assistance with low-interest loans, and direct subsidies, for examples, or linking payments to technology utilization. These measures also apply to other countries such as Canada and the U.K, where providers would still have to purchase their own healthcare ICT. As we have noted all along, the cumulative benefits of healthcare ICT implementation would help us achieve our dual healthcare delivery goals. However, these technologies need to be implemented by all healthcare stakeholders to a greater or lesser extent depending on which stakeholder, and their needs. In other words, we need to promote the implementation and use of these technologies across board, including among healthcare consumers. We need to let the word out about the gains derivable from these technologies to all constituencies. The healthcare consumer would able to communicate with the provider if the former had some rudimentary healthcare ICT capabilities, which are in place in many countries, developed and developing already, for example, the Internet, and even the cell phone. In particular, in order to be able to manage seniors at home, which is possible, and in fact could be more efficient and cost-effective via healthcare ICT, there would have to be some connectivity between the seniors and their healthcare providers. We do not expect all seniors to be able to operate sophisticated technologies, but software vendors and healthcare ICT manufacturers recognize the vast markets and are indeed already developing a variety of assistive technologies tailor-made for seniors that could facilitate the monitoring of seniors health conditions such as diabetes, high blood pressure and many other chronic diseases. We should also be focusing on developing cutting-edge healthcare ICT for operating community and ambulatory, besides domiciliary healthcare delivery in anticipation of the increase in the numbers of seniors in the years ahead. Many doctors are already using a computer with a videoconferencing link to treat their patients living for example in remote and rural areas, many of these patients, elderly. Several doctors in Spain, Italy, and Denmark are now using a telecounselling service that HEALTHOPTIMUM developed in 2005 according to a recent IST Results report. The project, funded under the EC's eTEN programme is helping to trigger the telemedicine deployment across Europe. HEALTH OPTIMUM solutions are Internet-based and work along with a telelaboratory service that enables the remote analysis of patient test samples, with remarkable benefits on healthcare delivery reported where implemented, including doctors saving time, public healthcare systems saving money by obviating the need for hospital visits and stays, and patients receiving improved quality, convenient, and well-coordinated healthcare. Besides saving the patients the trouble of traveling to the hospital to see a specialist, they could see him/her via videoconference with their family doctors in attendance, making for better service coordination, as the family doctor or GP and the specialist could jointly review patient data, including scans and lab investigations, via the telecounselling service. What's more, the results are quantifiable, facilitating quality evaluation and assurance. One trial used this service to connect primary healthcare facilities to hospital neurology departments, enabling the accurate assessment and diagnosis of patients with head injuries, without the need to transfer the patient to a hospital, which essentially exemplifies what we have been discussing that the use of appropriate healthcare ICT could help us achieve the dual objectives mentioned earlier. Indeed, the service in this trial led to almost 80%

reduction in the number of people referred to a specialist facility, with no doubt substantial cost savings, in a situation where previously would mean referring 53% of these patients, but only 11% now were. There was in fact improvement rather than depreciation in the quality of care in this trial because the diagnosis was reliable as the neurologist had access to scans and data from the primary healthcare facility, the patient also prevented from unwarranted and unanticipated risk that could result from moving the patient from place to place. When there is need for such transfers and surgery, the telecounselling system enables doctors to access information about the patient in advance, hence to prepare more swiftly and efficiently for the procedure. The systems telelaboratory analysis capabilities also help facilitate patient management with the potential to save lives. Primary healthcare providers could obtain samples of a patient's blood or urine for examples, remotely, analyze them on the spot, at the patient's home or bedside, and transmit the results to a specialist wirelessly, over a secure Public Key Infrastructure (PKI), the results obtained/sent back within ten minutes in most cases, processes that might have taken days. Does this not underscore the crucial role that healthcare ICT could play in process improvement and the need for us to promote the widespread implementation and utilization of these technologies? Should other countries and health jurisdiction not employ such technologies by developing their own or collaborating with the HEALTH OPTIMUM project for adaptation and expansion of these valuable technologies, as is the case now in Europe with trials expected in Sweden and Romania, among other countries in the near future? There is no doubt that these technologies will serve the anticipated increased health service needs of the increasingly aging populations in these countries very well. In particular, there would be increasing demand on the health systems of many countries developed or developing, for community/ambulatory and domiciliary health services that such telemedicine technologies would facilitate cost-effectively, as lower tax revenues due to a relative decline in the number of young people entering the labor market results increasingly in budget tightening. We need to brace up for the tasks ahead as changes in the health climate loom. Healthcare ICT could help prepare us adequately for these imminent new times.

References

1. Wald A, Kamm MA, Müller-Lissner SA, Scarpignato C, Marx W, Schuijt C. The BI Omnibus Study: An international survey of community prevalence of constipation and laxative use in adults. Digestive Disorders Week. 20-25 May 2006.

2. Müller-Lissner SA, Kamm MA, Scarpignato C, Wald A. Myths and Misconceptions About Chronic Constipation. *American Journal of Gastroenterology* 2005; 100(1):232-42.

3. Available at: http://www.phac-aspc.gc.ca/ccdpc-cpcmc/bc-cds/publications/reduce_e.html
Accessed on May 30, 2006

4. Miller, R.H., West, C., & Tiffany Martin Brown et al., The Value of Electronic Health Records in Solo or Small Group Practices *Health Affairs*, September/October 2005, 24 (5): 1127⁻37

5. Kaushal, R. et al. (2005) The Costs of a National Health Information Network. *Annals of Internal Medicine* 143, 165-173.

6. Walker, J. (2005) The Value of Health Care Information Exchange and Interoperability. *Health Affairs* Web exclusive. Published Jan. 19.

Conclusion

We have attempted to discuss some of the salient issues concerning healthcare delivery today, in particular as they apply to the provision of qualitative health services to seniors at affordable costs. There is no doubt about the general applicability of our contention that healthcare delivery is a conglomeration of processes and that to achieve our dual objectives of delivering qualitative healthcare and reducing healthcare spending at the same time, we need to decompose and understand how these processes work singly and in tandem with one another. We have seen in the e-book the need for us to do this not just for fancy but also as being imperative. We have pointed to the soaring healthcare spending among nations, which none of them could afford in the long term, even if only on the perfectly reasonable ground that resources, in particular financial resources, are limited, and must dwindle with continuing and ever-increasing use, for example on healthcare expenditures. There is no doubt that this would be the case as countries spend ever more of their total economic output on health. Interestingly, there is evidence that such increased health spending does not necessarily translate into better quality healthcare delivery. In fact, the relationship could be reciprocal in some instances. So, then, what is the rationale in spending so much on healthcare when in fact the health of the people on which we expend these enormous resources worsen rather than improve? This anomalous situation alone is enough reason to figure that there is a mismatch somewhere in the healthcare delivery chain. It clearly indicates that we are doing something wrong somewhere along the line toward our final output, which is thus flawed. Invariably, what we are doing wrong is not appreciating that healthcare delivery is a cacophony of processes that need proper alignment for a perfect or near-perfect outcome. There are of course a variety of ways by which we could approach the matter but healthcare ICT, appropriately deployed offers us an efficient and cost-effective way to ensure this proper alignment, improve the efficiency and effectiveness of the processes, hence the quality of the final outcome, namely healthcare delivery, while reducing transactions costs. Since the transactional basis of the underlying processes holds for any health system, regardless of its funding model, or its other peculiarities, for example, physician recompense model, and since no model could claim to be perfect, and could indeed never be, we argue that every health system needs to embark on this process decomposition exercise. It should not alarm anyone that a health system could never be perfect considering the dynamic nature of the innumerable variables that are the keystones health, healthcare, and the health system. In fact, as we discussed in this e-book, we need to embrace these changes, as they constitute the fodder for our continuous quality improvement exercises. They not only challenge us to address the problems that they pose threatening to make us lose the gains we have so far made in improving the quality of our healthcare delivery, but also reveal to us the preparations we need to make in anticipation of projected perhaps even imminent issues and problems that could pose a similar threat. In other words, our process decomposition exercise reveals newer, some perhaps even cryptic processes that we need to improve now, and down the road to keep our health services up to mark, and to ensure resource optimization, hence save healthcare costs. This process would yield even newer facts based on even newer changes, and the quality improvement processes continue ad infinitum.

In both publicly funded and privately funded health systems, the public sectors

provide most of the funds for health service provision, and indeed, the money that individuals earn to survive and to maintain their families, out which an increasing amount goes into payments for healthcare services. Thus, in the U.S, federal compensation has grown a lot faster than private compensation lately a 115% versus 69% increase respectively, since 1990, in the government and private sectors, the average wages, increased to 104% and 65% in the government and private sectors respectively. The U.S. Bureau of Economic Analysis data show for example that the average federal worker earned $100,178 in wages and benefits in 2004, compared to $51,876 for the average private-sector worker, and for averages alone, federal workers earned an average $66,558, 56% more than the $42,635 of the average private worker. Indeed, the private sector is also reducing other benefits, in particular, health benefits, as many claim, as a crucial measure to remain solvent let alone, profitable. Many are also offering employees early retirement packages, and others embracing a variety of cost-sharing health plans. With healthcare costs increasing and likely to increase even more with the anticipated increase in the number of seniors in the years ahead, there is no doubt about the incredible financial burden that the private sector would increasingly bear. This would result in either healthcare costs etching an increasing chunk of the gross domestic product, with implications for the provision of other services, or government raising the money from taxpayers via higher taxes, among other means. With higher taxes for example, would be less discretionary income, including with which to pay for healthcare, even in publicly funded health systems such as in Canada where individuals still need private insurance for some health services that Medicare does not cover. This might mean some people forgoing those services, many of which are crucial to some people's well being, for example, dental care, if not even their very survival, for example, vision care. The result would be many more people becoming ill, further increasing the financial burden on the health system, not to mention the financial, physical, and emotional burden on the ill individual and his/her family. Thus, besides the fact that every system needs ongoing

245

process improvement and quality assurance, they also face perennial costs constraints as different services compete for limited resources. Costs are also significant handicaps to the adoption of healthcare ICT by the end-user. The onus is therefore on us to continue to seek ways to ensure that our health systems do not collapse or for that matter our economies. Simultaneously, we need to continue to promote the widespread diffusion and utilization of healthcare ICT as these technologies have the potential to help us achieve our dual goals of improving healthcare delivery while saving costs. We need to continue to address the issues standing in the way of the pervasive diffusion and utilization of these technologies, lest we miss the opportunities for exploiting their immense benefits. The factors that determine the success or other wise of our efforts intertwine intricately, and our approach should bear this in mind, adapted of course to our particular health system. We need to consider for example if and to what extent we should offer healthcare providers incentives to purchase healthcare ICT. In ensuring that they have, a stake in these technologies hence would want to make them work, should we ignore the urgency in encouraging the pervasive diffusion of these technologies in helping us achieve the dual objectives of qualitative healthcare delivery at affordable costs, or should we not? Each country has to answer questions such as these based on important local monetary and other determinants, recognizing for example that some jurisdictions might not have the resources to finance such incentives and would have to devise others means to encourage its providers to invest in these technologies. Each jurisdiction would likely face other peculiar challenges. These challenges as we have seen in our discussion thus far are many, and range from technical, to legal, to clinical, and even to ethico-moral challenges. Nonetheless, we need to tackle each of them until resolved, as our hopes of solving the problems our health systems face, hinge on such resolutions. We would for example still not achieve the dual objectives implementing these technologies but with none utilizing them. In other words, even if we implemented the infrastructure for a regional health information network (RHIN), we need to encourage healthcare providers to purchase the healthcare ICT that they need to hook up with the network, and indeed, to utilize these technologies, not just for basic tasks and transactions, but for quality assurance activities as well. Would we, either with legislation lacking to back up e-prescriptions, or the handling of patient data to ensure their privacy and confidentiality, for examples? On May 22, 2006, the U.S Department of Veterans Affairs (VA) announced the theft from the residence of a VA employee, unauthorized to take the storage medium home in the first place, of personal data on 26.5 million U.S. veterans. The data in the laptop and disc lost included names, social security numbers, and dates of birth, among others, for the veterans, and in many cases for their spouses, leaving them exposed to identity theft. Now a coalition of consumer privacy groups in the health care industry is requesting the U.S. Department of Health and Human Services (DHHS) to conduct a Health Insurance Portability and Accountability Act, 1996 (HIPAA) compliance review of the VA after this unprecedented and extensive security breach. Would such a law if properly applied not improve processes at VA eventually? On the other hand, some critics of the U.S. health savings plans (HSA), an insurance option commenced in 2004, contend that too rigid rules bog down the program, compromising its effectiveness. They argue for example that HSA, essentially tax-preferred savings account plus high-deductible health insurance, favors the rich and healthy, for whom affording the high deductibles, is easier. HSA critics argue that rather than help minimize the effect of government over the consumer's choices by reducing the price distortions due to the federal tax code, it does the exact opposite, the HSA law giving the consumer less leeway to make vital healthcare choices, and those with chronic illnesses to put away funds for projected healthcare expenses, among others. These issues have led to calls for government to review the HSA, for example as President plans to do increasing the limits to savings and tax credits, but also to expand the program, with the consumer ultimately fully in control of his/her funds. Both instances of the applications of legislation to healthcare delivery however, illustrate the point about healthcare delivery being an assemblage of processes, which by improving, via healthcare ICT appropriately deployed for example would necessarily improve healthcare delivery.

To illustrate this point, let us consider one critical aspect of the process

improvement efforts that healthcare ICT could help us achieve effectively and efficiently, namely, to rectify the current pervasive health information asymmetry in the health industry. One of the handicaps to the success of the HSA as mentioned above is the healthcare consumer not having enough room to maneuver regarding taking proper healthcare decisions. One of the main reasons for this is because of the information asymmetry mentioned above. How could we expect the healthcare consumer for example to make the most rational choice of healthcare provider not having any information by which to go? This explains the wisdom in the publication online by the U.S government on June 1, 2006 of how much Medicare pays for hip replacements, cardiac surgery, and 28 other procedures in each of the country's counties, part of the plan to make such public knowledge of hospital price information routine, eventually. This move would certainly also please employers and other payers of the country's $1.9 trillion health care bill, but government needs to follow it up with the release of other relevant pricing and healthcare quality data and information. The public could view this information on the Centers for Medicare and Medicaid Services (CMS) website, which already also has some quality data. However, government should also take its efforts a step further by delivering this and other relevant information via targeted, and contextualized healthcare ICT-backed, health information dissemination, as many people might not even know that the information on the website is out and there, let alone where to find it. This latter point illustrates what we have been saying in this e-book about decomposing processes and addressing revealed issues at each decomposition stage, thereby moving closer to further process improvement, in this case, rectifying the information asymmetry on pricing, which posting the information on the CMS web site might not fully achieve. To be sure, Medicare officials hinted at releasing the information being an initial step in a planned broad effort by both the government and the private sector to publish price and quality informat ion to its about 43 million elderly and disabled beneficiaries. Notably however is that in the private sector, relatively few insurers released limited cost and quality information to their members, a process that clearly needs improving if we were to achieve our goal of providing the health consumer the information required to make informed decisions based on an objective comparison of hospitals and doctors on cost, quality and consumer approval. Critics of the newly released information have pointed to its limited value to healthcare consumers because the data lack hospital-specific pricing information, and that on payments private insurance or the uninsured might make, although it has that Medicare does, even then not what individual Medicare member pays. These observations again mean that the information posted on the CMS website does not fully rectify the information asymmetry that it should, hence the need for additional process improvements to reduce the adverse consequences on the entire health system that such deficiencies could engender. This also highlights the need to utilize fully, the healthcare technologies that we implement lest we would be denying ourselves of their full benefits, and the chances to recoup our investments on them in both material and human terms. As we have emphasized in our discussion, the issue of the healthcare consumer having the necessary health information to make important healthcare decisions is one we need to take seriously, as information asymmetry could derail all our efforts to improve the quality of healthcare delivery. As also mentioned earlier, we should actually endeavor to deliver this information to those individuals that need them utilizing cost-effective and efficient health information technologies. Besides general health information and on new research findings then, we could also use these technologies to deliver treatment information that could facilitate disease resolution. Would it not for example speed up the cure of a bacterial infection of the urethra text messaging the results of the laboratory analysis of a mid-stream urine specimen to a patient via his/her cell phone as well as instructions to pick up the required prescription of antibiotics that the doctor has also sent to the pharmacy electronically? Would this not save both the patient a trip to the hospital, and the doctor, precious time he/she could use treating another perhaps more ill patient? Do these questions not also underscore the importance of process improvement in healthcare delivery, and how healthcare ICT could help us achieve this goal? Our discussion in this e-book clearly indicates that we have many opportunities to improve the quality of our healthcare delivery simultaneously reducing health spending. The choice now is ours to tap the resources that the widespread diffusion and utilization of healthcare ICT offer. There is no doubt that we would continue in our present efforts to do so knowing that the future of our health services, and of our ability to meet the healthcare needs of our seniors and indeed, of every member of society rests squarely on the efforts to continue to pursue our goals vigorously and with utmost determination to succeed.